Developmental Psychopathology at School

Series Editors:
Shane R. Jimerson

Stephen E. Brock

For further volumes:
http://www.springer.com/series/7495

Huijun Li · Melissa Pearrow · Shane R. Jimerson

Identifying, Assessing, and Treating Early Onset Schizophrenia at School

Springer

Huijun Li
Department of Public Psychiatry,
Commonwealth Research Center
Harvard Medical School
Beth Israel Deaconess Medical Center
Boston, MA
USA
hli5@bidmc.harvard.edu

Melissa Pearrow
Department of Counseling and
School Psychology
University of Massachusetts
Wheatley Hall 2-169
Boston, MA
USA
melissa.pearrow@umb.edu

Shane R. Jimerson
Gevirtz Graduate School of Education
Department of Counseling,
Clinical, and School Psychology
University of California
Santa Barbara
USA
jimerson@education.uscb.edu

ISBN 978-1-4419-6271-3 e-ISBN 978-1-4419-6272-0
DOI 10.1007/978-1-4419-6272-0
Springer New York Dordrecht Heidelberg London

Library of Congress Control Number: 2010934366

Printed on acid-free paper

Springer is part of Springer Science+Business Media (www.springer.com)

This book is dedicated to youth, their families, and the professionals who persist and overcome the profound challenges associated with early onset schizophrenia.

It is our aim to bring science to practice, with the intent of enhancing the development of youth and contributing important information to the efforts of families and professionals.

And also to our children and families who inspire us and remind us of the importance of our efforts each day:

Weiwen Li	*Mark Pearrow*	*Gavin Jimerson*
Yue Li	*Eleanor Pearrow*	*Taite Jimerson*
	Jason Pearrow	*Kathryn O'Brien*

Acknowledgments

In any project of this scope, we believe it important to acknowledge the contributions of the individuals who contributed to our efforts. First, Dr. Li would like to acknowledge the great mentorship of Drs. Larry Seidman, Matcheri Keshavan, Margarita Alegria, and Regina Yando in my professional development. I would also like to thank my colleagues at the Commonwealth Research Center, Drs Joanne Wojcik, Anthony Giuliano, Michelle Friedman-Yakoobian, and Raquelle Mesholam-Gately; and Ms Maryan Picard for their tremendous support in my transition to a new research field. Dr. Pearrow would like to acknowledge both Drs. Virginia Harvey and Lisa Cosgrove for their wisdom and guidance in linking scholarly work with the communities that are impacted by it. She also would like to acknowledge Janet Powell, Peggy Farren, and NSPC for their living examples of kind, supportive and effective treatments with vulnerable children and families. Dr. Jimerson would like to acknowledge the outstanding graduate students with whom he has the good fortune to collaborate with daily. He would also like to acknowledge Dr. Byron Egeland and Dr. Alan Sroufe of the Institute of Child Development at the University of Minnesota for their important contributions to his preparation and understanding of developmental psychopathology, developmental trajectories, and engaging in scholarly activities that promote the well-being of children and families.

Contents

Chapter 1
Introduction

Early Onset Schizophrenia (EOS, onset of symptoms prior to age 18 years) is the diagnostic classification identifying children and adolescents experiencing delusions (having beliefs not based on reality), hallucinations (seeing or hearing things that do not exist), disorganized or incoherent speech, grossly disorganized or catatonic behavior or negative symptoms such as lack of emotion (American Psychiatric Association [APA], 2000). It has been estimated that about one in 10,000 children will develop some form of schizophrenic disorder, with childhood-onset schizophrenia (COS, onset prior to age 12 years) occurring in roughly one in 40,000 children (Asarnow & Asarnow, 2003; Nicolson & Rapoport, 1999; Remschmidt, 2002). Mueser and McGurk (2004) report a lifetime prevalence of Schizophrenia to be one in 100, and it is estimated that 2.5 million people in the United States are living with the disorder. The symptomology required for diagnosis is considered to be the same as for adults. Most frequently, the age of onset of schizophrenia is between 16 and 35 years old (Asarnow, Thompson, & McGrath, 2004).

There is evidence that EOS is very similar to adult onset schizophrenia. However, over the course of development the disorder is often more severe than adult onset schizophrenia (Asarnow et al., 2004; Kumra & Schulz, 2008). Importantly, when schizophrenia develops during childhood or adolescence, the symptoms impact the individual as well as his or her family, peers, teachers, and other school professionals. While relatively rare, it is imperative that school psychologists and other mental health professionals working in the schools are well informed about EOS so that they are fully prepared to meet the needs of these students. Therefore, a thorough knowledge of EOS is crucial to increase the likelihood of success in all domains of their lives.

Why School Professionals Should Read This Book

The importance of understanding EOS is that its effects are among the most pervasive and debilitating of all childhood psychopathologies. Of notable significance in the educational context, schizophrenia is associated with impairments in cognitive abilities, language skills, motor skills, social skills, and creative thought, among

H. Li et al., *Identifying, Assessing, and Treating Early Onset Schizophrenia at School*, Developmental Psychopathology at School, DOI 10.1007/978-1-4419-6272-0_1,

other domains (Andreasen, 2000; Nicolson et al., 2000; Remschmidt, 2002). Moreover, the early identification of EOS will facilitate early intervention designed to address the needs of the student. Furthermore, how and where to serve students with EOS are difficult questions. Some students with EOS may need to be served in alternative or special education settings and others in general education settings. To appropriately address the needs of all children and to address public perceptions, school psychologists and other educational professionals need to be prepared to identify, assess, and treat students with EOS in the school setting. In this section, we review some key issues regarding the importance of identifying and addressing the needs of students with EOS.

Students with EOS face numerous challenges at school. EOS is associated with behaviors that interfere with school success, including cognitive and social skill deficits. These deficits may also be associated with poor peer relationships and low academic achievement. Problem behaviors common among students with EOS include, social withdrawal, isolation, disruptive behavior disorders, problems paying attention, impaired memory and reasoning, inappropriate or flattened expression of emotion, achievement difficulties, speech and language problems, and developmental delays (McClellan et al., 2003). Behaviors associated with EOS may result in discipline referrals and at times result in suspension and/or expulsion from school. As a result of the challenges they face at school, many students with EOS will meet special education eligibility criteria.

Inclusion of children with EOS in general education classrooms. Students with disabilities are increasingly placed in general education settings (Smith, 2007). Given that support services may be offered in both the general or special educational settings regardless of eligibility status, it is typical that educational professionals across both contexts will be responsible for facilitating their education. Hence, all educational professionals (in both special and general education) need to have up-to-date information on EOS.

Importance of early identification and intervention. Early identification and intervention are important components influencing developmental trajectories of students with EOS. Identifying risk factors and recognizing early signs are important steps in supporting students with EOS. The premorbid abnormalities and early onset of psychotic symptoms found in children with schizophrenia often lead to a severe disruption in the child's global development. Skill deficits in numerous domains often exist due to the child's inability to develop or acquire new skills during the early stages of the disorder; hence the importance of early identification.

EOS is typically identified during the school-age years. Research reveals that the rate of schizophrenic disorders escalates during adolescence, between the ages of 13 and 17 years (Remschmidt, 2002). Thus, educational professionals across the middle and high school years must be knowledgeable and prepared to identify symptoms, and to provide support services. Research reveals that individuals whose first onset of schizophrenia occurred before the age of 13 years had much greater premorbid, language, motor, social delay, academic (e.g., either failed a grade or required placement in special education) deficits, and overall poor neuropsychological functioning in attention, working memory and executive function compared to those individuals with onset occurring during later adolescence (Giedd et al., 1999; Nicolson et al., 2000), these data suggest that there is an opportunity for early identification. The first step in supporting students is understanding and recognizing risk factors and early indicators in early and middle childhood.

School-based professionals have daily opportunities to support students. Most youths with EOS attend school. Thus, there is an opportunity to establish support services to help facilitate the development of these students. For those children who continue to attend school, educational professionals are in a unique position to help facilitate adaptive behaviors and life skills that not only help them be more successful in school, but also serve as a foundation for adult living.

EOS is frequently experienced concurrently with other problems. Roughly two-thirds of children who meet the diagnostic criteria for EOS also meet criteria for other mental disorders (House, 1999). EOS has most often been diagnosed concurrently with oppositional/conduct disorder (31%) and atypical depression/dysthymic disorder (37%; Asarnow & Asarnow, 2003). Furthermore, differential diagnoses of EOS is especially difficult due to similar symptoms with classifications such autism and pervasive developmental disorder (Eggers, Bunk, & Krause, 2000).

Education and learning are important for future success. Low achievement, truancy, and school drop out are each associated with poorer outcomes as young adults. For students with EOS, facilitating and maintaining student engagement in the educational process help to provide these students with the skills and knowledge that may benefit them in the future. In addition, educational successes promote subsequent healthy adaptation and adjustment. Unfortunately, research reveals that individuals with schizophrenia and paranoid delusional disorder are markedly less likely to work during adulthood (Zwerling et al., 2002).

Mandated by federal legislation. It is important to note that section 504 of the *Rehabilitation Act of 1973* articulates the provision of special services to ensure that students with disabilities receive a free and appropriate public education (FAPE). According to Section 504, a qualified student is defined as any person who has a mental or physical impairment that substantially limits a major life activity (e.g., learning). Thus, depending upon the manifestation of symptoms and impairment of functioning, children with EOS *may* or *may not* qualify under Section 504 (see Table 1.1 for further details). Thus, students thought to have EOS should be evaluated to determine whether they qualify for services.

Under the new *Individuals with Disability Improvement Act (IDEIA, 2004)*, if a special education student has a disciplinary plan, and receives a disciplinary referral, the team must investigate and determine if the student's actions were a direct result of his or her disability. It is important to note that the education classification of Emotional Disturbance (ED) specifically includes schizophrenia (the IDEIA definition of ED is included in Table 1.2). For the student with EOS, who also meets special education eligibility criteria, school districts must ensure that disciplinary procedures do not interfere with the provision of a free and appropriate public education. IDEIA directs the Individualized Education Program (IEP) team to focus on addressing behavioral problems of children with disabilities to enhance their success in the classroom. For instance, in IDEIA, it is specifically delineated that

Table 1.1 Summary Regarding Section 504 Coverage of Children with Early Onset Schizophrenia

QUESTION: What is Early Onset Schizophrenia? *ANSWER*: Early Onset Schizophrenia (onset prior to the age of 18 years) is the diagnostic classification identifying children and adolescents experiencing delusions (having beliefs not based on reality), hallucinations (seeing or hearing things that do not exist), disorganized or incoherent speech, grossly disorganized or catatonic behavior or negative symptoms such as lack of emotion (DSM-IV-TR, 2000).
QUESTION: Are all children with EOS automatically protected under Section 504? *ANSWER*: NO. Some children with EOS may have a disability within the meaning of Section 504; others may not. Children must meet the Section 504 definition of disability to be protected under the regulation. Under Section 504, a "person with disabilities" is defined as any person who has a physical or mental impairment which substantially limits a major life activity (e.g., learning). Thus, depending on the severity of their condition, children with EOS may or may not fit within that definition.
QUESTION: Must children thought to have EOS be evaluated by school districts? *ANSWER*: YES. If parents believe that their child has a disability, whether it be EOS or any other impairment, and the school district has reason to believe that the child may need special education or related services, the school district must evaluate the child. If the school district does not believe the child needs special education or related services, and thus does not evaluate the child, the school district must notify the parents of their due process rights.
QUESTION: Must school districts have a different evaluation process for Section 504 and the IDEIA? *ANSWER*: NO. School districts may use the same process for evaluating the needs of students under Section 504 that they use for implementing IDEIA.
QUESTION: Can school districts have a different evaluation process for Section 504? *ANSWER*: YES. School districts may have a separate process for evaluating the needs of students under Section 504. However, they must follow the requirements for evaluation specified in the Section 504 regulation.
QUESTION: Is a child with EOS, who has a disability within the meaning of Section 504 but not under the IDEIA, entitled to receive special education services? *ANSWER*: YES and NO. If a child with EOS is found to have a disability within the meaning of Section 504, he or she may receive any special education services the placement team decides to be necessary; however, he or she is entitled to either regular or special education services that provide an education comparable to that provided to students without disabilities.
QUESTION: Can a school district refuse to provide special education services to a child with EOS because he or she does not meet the eligibility criteria under the IDEIA? *ANSWER*: YES and NO. School districts are only required to provide special education services to anyone who is identified. They can, however, provide services to nonidentified youngsters if they wish to do so. Alternately, they may provide regular education accommodations to ensure that the student's education is comparable to that provided to students without disabilities.
QUESTION: Can a child with EOS, who is protected under Section 504, receive related aids and services in the regular educational setting? *ANSWER*: YES. Should it be determined that a child with EOS has a disability within the meaning of Section 504 and needs only adjustments in the regular classroom, rather than special education, those adjustments are required by Section 504.
QUESTION: Can parents request a due process hearing if a school district refuses to evaluate their child for EOS? *ANSWER*: YES. In fact, parents may request a due process hearing to challenge any actions regarding the identification, evaluation, or educational placement of their child with a disability, whom they believe needs special education or related services.

(continued)

Table 1.1 (continued)

QUESTION: Must a school district have a separate hearing procedure for Section 504 and the IDEI A?

ANSWER: NO. School districts may use the same procedures for resolving disputes under both Section 504 and the IDEIA. In fact, many local school districts and some state education agencies are conserving time and resources by using the same due process procedures. However, education agencies should ensure that hearing officers are knowledgeable about the requirements of Section 504.

QUESTION: Can school districts use separate due process procedures for Section 504?

ANSWER: YES. School districts may have a separate system of procedural safeguards in place to resolve Section 504 disputes. However, these procedures must follow the requirements of the Section 504 regulation.

QUESTION: What should parents do if the state hearing process does not include Section 504?

ANSWER: Under Section 504, school districts are required to provide procedural safeguards and inform parents of these procedures. Thus, school districts are responsible for providing a Section 504 hearing even if the State process does not include it.

Note: The above is a modification of the 1993 Memorandum from the United States Department of Education regarding: Clarification of School Districts' Responsibilities to Evaluate Children with Attention Deficit Disorders (ADD). The original document focused exclusively on ADD; however, the information would also be applicable to Early Onset Schizophrenia (EOS).

Table 1.2 Individuals with Disabilities Education Improvement Act (2004) Definition of Demotional Disturbance

The term (Emotional Disturbance) means a condition exhibiting one or more of the following characteristics over a long period of time and to a marked degree that adversely affects a child's educational performance:

1. An inability to learn that cannot be explained by intellectual, sensory, or health factors
2. An inability to build or maintain satisfactory interpersonal relationships with peers and teachers
3. Inappropriate types of behavior or feelings under normal circumstances
4. A general pervasive mood of unhappiness or depression
5. A tendency to develop physical symptoms or fears associated with personal or school problems

The term includes schizophrenia. The term does not apply to children who are socially maladjusted, unless it is determined that they have an emotional disturbance

(a) the IEP team explore the need for strategies and support systems to address any behavior that may impede the learning of the child with the disability or the learning of his or her peers and (b) that the school districts shall address the in-service and preservice personnel needs (including those of professionals and paraprofessionals who provide special education, general education, related services, or early intervention services) as they relate to developing and implementing positive intervention strategies. Thus, it is imperative that both general and special education professionals be prepared to provide educational services to students with EOS.

In addition, the *Americans with Disabilities Act of 1990* (ADA) and recently enacted *Americans with Disabilities Act Amendments Act (ADAAA)* also apply to students with EOS, as ADA prohibits discrimination against persons with disabilities at work (Gioia & Brekke, 2003), at school and in public accommodations, and also applies to institutions that do not receive federal funds. Because ADA has been interpreted as incorporating many of the Section 504 requirements, it has been suggested that by meeting 504 requirements, school districts fulfill their ADA obligations (Soleil, 2000). Furthermore, meeting IDEIA requirements also fulfills 504 requirements.

Early Onset Schizophrenia Diagnostic Criteria

Diagnostic criteria for Schizophrenia and Other Psychotic Disorders are delineated in the *Diagnostic and Statistical Manual of Mental Disorders* (Text Rev, 4th ed.; DSM IV-TR; APA, 2000); the classifications are included in Fig. 1.1. The following provides a brief summary of the criteria according to the *DSM IV-TR* (Chapter 5 delineates the full criteria). Diagnostic characteristics of schizophrenia include: delusions (i.e., having beliefs not based on reality), hallucinations (i.e., seeing or hearing things that do not exist), disorganized speech, grossly disorganized or catatonic behavior, and negative symptoms (i.e., affective flattening). A diagnosis is appropriate when two of the preceding are present during a 1-month period, and symptoms persist for at least six months. When the onset is prior to the age of 18 years, it is considered as Early Onset Schizophrenia. There are five subtypes of schizophrenia:

1. *Paranoid-type* schizophrenia is characterized by delusions and auditory hallucinations.
2. *Disorganized-type* schizophrenia is characterized by speech and behavior that are disorganized or difficult to understand, and flattening or inappropriate emotions.

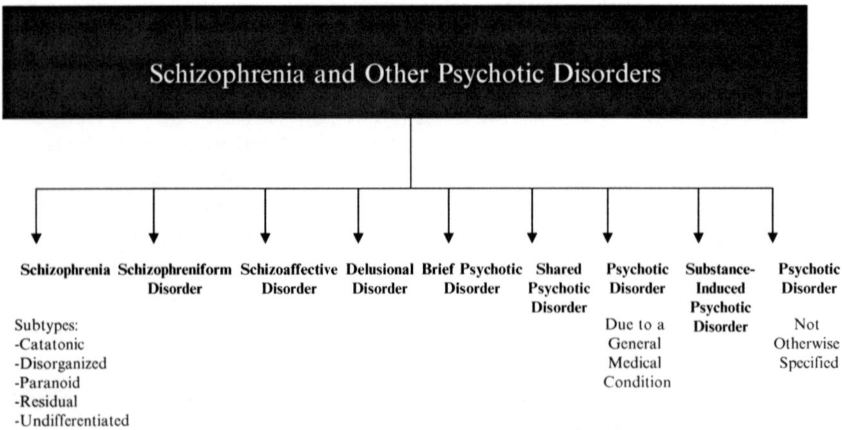

Fig. 1.1 Nine Categories of Schizophrenia and Other Psychotic Disorders

Table 1.3 Brief Summary of Other Psychotic Classifications

Schizophreniform disorder. Is characterized by the same symptoms of schizophrenia, however, the distinction is the duration, in that symptoms last more than one month but less than six months.
Schizoaffective disorder. Is the classification when individuals present with symptoms of both schizophrenia and a mood disorder (i.e., unipolar depression or bipolar disorder).
Delusional disorder. People with this illness have nonbizarre delusions (e.g., beliefs of something occurring in a person's life which is not out of the realm of possibility) that persist for at least one month, but no other symptoms characteristic of schizophrenia.
Brief psychotic disorder. People with this illness have sudden, short periods of psychotic behavior, often in response to a very stressful event (e.g., death in the family).
Shared psychotic disorder. This diagnosis is applicable when a person develops delusions in the context of a relationship with another person who already has his or her own delusion(s). Children can be particularly vulnerable to this given their inter-dependency in early development.
Psychotic disorder due to a medical condition. This classification is used when hallucinations, delusions, or other symptoms are the result of another illness that affects brain function, such as a head injury or brain tumor.
Substance-induced psychotic disorder. This condition is caused by the use of or withdrawal from some substances (e.g., alcohol, cocaine), that may cause hallucinations, delusions, or confused speech.
Psychotic disorder – not otherwise specified. This classification includes psychotic symptomatology (i.e., delusions, hallucinations, disorganized speech, grossly disorganized, or catatonic behavior), however, it is used when there is inadequate information to make a specific diagnosis.

Note: see DSM IV-TR (APA, 2000) for a complete review of all diagnostic criteria.

3. *Catatonic-type* schizophrenia is characterized by disturbances of movement (e.g., grossly disorganized or immobility).
4. *Undifferentiated-type* schizophrenia is characterized by some symptoms seen in the other subtypes of schizophrenia, but not enough of any one of them to define it as another particular type of schizophrenia.
5. *Residual-type* schizophrenia is characterized by a past history of at least one episode of schizophrenia, but the person currently has no positive symptoms (delusions, hallucinations, disorganized speech, or behavior).

The other psychotic disorders classifications are briefly described in Table 1.3.

EOS and Educational Support Services

As is the case for all *DSM* diagnostic categories, meeting the *DSM IV-TR* (APA, 2000) criteria for schizophrenia *does not* necessarily qualify a student for special educational placement and/or related services. Depending upon the severity of a student's EOS, a student *may* be considered eligible for services and/or related aids under Section 504 of the *Rehabilitation Act of 1973* or *IDEIA* (2004). The following section provides a discussion of educational regulations that govern the provision of special services to ensure that the student with EOS receives a free and appropriate public education (FAPE).

If a student with EOS is judged to be eligible (see Table 1.1 for a discussion of relevant considerations), then Section 504 of the *Rehabilitation Act of 1973* emphasizes that the individual is entitled to a FAPE. This may include either regular or special education-related aids and services (Davila, Williams, & MacDonald, 1991). One way to fulfill the FAPE mandate is to provide an Individualized Education Program (IEP), although it is not required under Section 504. If special education services are not appropriate for the student with EOS (and the student is judged to be a "handicapped person" as described by Section 504), then appropriate support services should be provided in the general education setting. Furthermore, it is important to note that general education classroom teachers are essential in the identification of required instructional adaptations and interventions. The accommodations for students eligible under Section 504 need to be individualized to be effective; thus, there is no single plan that will fit the needs of each student.

If a student with EOS is found to qualify for special education services according to *IDEIA* (2004), then that individual would receive specially designed instruction, at no cost to his or her parents, to meet the unique needs of the child with a disability. Under the protection of special education, the child with EOS has the right to: (a) procedural safeguards to ensure that parents are provided a written notice regarding identification, evaluation, and/or placement, or any change in placement of their child in special education, (b) a comprehensive evaluation by a multidisciplinary team focused on serving the child in the least restrictive environment (LRE), and (c) impartial due process hearing for parents who disagree with the identification, evaluation, or placement of a child. In many instances, students diagnosed with EOS may qualify for special education under the eligibility category of emotional disturbance, while others may not qualify as they may not reach diagnostic threshold (e.g., behaviors do not interfere with their learning or the learning of others) or their behavior difficulties are better described as socially maladjustment (SM) (also see Table 1.1 for further discussion). In assessing the potential impact of EOS on learning opportunities and school performance, it is important to consider how the disorder impacts attendance, task and assignment completion, peer relationships and cooperation, as these factors may impact the learning of the student. Guidelines regarding how to determine special education eligibility are discussed in more detail in Chapter 6.

Purpose and Plan of This Book

This book provides school professionals, as well as other child mental health professionals, and parents, essential information needed to be better prepared to identify and address the needs of students with EOS. Chapter 2 provides a review of the multiple influences and etiological considerations characterizing the contemporary understanding of what may lead to the development of EOS. Chapter 3 describes the prevalence and related epidemiological information for EOS. Chapter 4 provides information addressing early risk factors and screening procedures for EOS. Chapter 5 details the assessments available to determine if EOS is present. Chapter 6 details the consideration of EOS symptoms for psychoeducational assessments and special education eligibility. Chapter 7 provides a summary of research examining the effectiveness of interventions for youth with EOS, as well as, implementation considerations for the school setting. Finally, the Resource Appendix provides a review of websites that contain valuable information. It is expected that this book will serve as a valuable resource in identifying, understanding, and addressing the needs of students with EOS.

Chapter 2
Causes

The exact nature of the etiological process of schizophrenia still remains elusive. Contemporary scholarship suggests that multiple factors contribute to the development of schizophrenia, including: (a) genes that cause structural brain deviations which make some individuals vulnerable to schizophrenia and (b) environmental factors such as negative prenatal and postnatal impacts and social stresses such as trauma and stigma. Furthermore, there may be an interaction or interplay between genetic vulnerability, neurobiological, and environmental factors that put a child or adolescent at the risk of developing schizophrenia.

Genetics

There is evidence that schizophrenia may be inheritable. Familial studies have indicated that parents of youth with EOS have higher rates of schizophrenia spectrum disorders than parents of patients with adult-onset illness and relatives of children and adolescents with ADHD (Margari et al., 2008; Nicolson et al., 2003). The risk of developing schizophrenia is about ten times higher if a first-degree relative has the illness. Among monozygotic (identical twins) twins of patients with schizophrenia, about 50% may develop the illness, and among dizygotic twins (fraternal twins) of patients with schizophrenia, about 10–15% have the illness. Also, 9% siblings of patients with schizophrenia may develop the illness, and 6% in half siblings. The approximate chance of developing schizophrenia in a child is 40% if both parents have the illness and 12% if one parent has it (Miller & Mason, 2002). In addition, when a biological child of individuals with schizophrenia is adopted, he or she has an elevated risk than the general population of developing schizophrenia, as expected for first degree relatives. Further, if one of the identical twins has schizophrenia, the children of both identical twins may have higher rates of schizophrenia (Fatemi & Folsom, 2009). Overall, the heritability estimates of schizophrenia are about 80–85% (Craddock, O'Donovan, & Owen, 2006).

Recent findings from behavioral genetic studies of schizophrenia indicate that the heritable vulnerability is unlikely to result from a single genetic locus or even a

H. Li et al., *Identifying, Assessing, and Treating Early Onset Schizophrenia at School*, Developmental Psychopathology at School, DOI 10.1007/978-1-4419-6272-0_2,

small number of genes, rather resulting from multiple genes acting in concert or many single susceptibility genes acting independently (Walker, Kestler, Bollini, & Hochman, 2004). Researchers using molecular genetic techniques (such as candidate gene analyses, genome scans, and linkage studies) have identified several specific genes [e.g., serotonin type 2a receptor (5-HT2a) gene responsible for learning and memory and the dopamine D3 receptor gene for cognitive and emotional functions] as contributing to the development of schizophrenia (Badner & Gershon, 2002; Mowry & Nancarrow, 2001). More studies are needed to replicate such findings. Table 2.1 shows more risk genes for schizophrenia. In addition, many genetic alterations are proposed to be responsible for this illness. According to Lupski (2008), examples of such genetic alternations include "gain or loss of large chunks of DNA known as copy-number variations (CNVs). ... DNA rearrangements involve duplications and deletions that can result in many characteristics, including inherited neurological diseases ..." (p. 178). Walker et al. (2004) reported an association between the microdeletion on chromosome 22q11 deletion and schizophrenia. Such deletion occurs in about 0.025% of the general population, and it is often associated with structural abnormalities on the face, head, and heart. About 25% of individuals with 22q11 deletion meet the diagnostic criteria of schizophrenia, and the rate of this deletion appears to be higher in individuals with EOS or COS. More recently, researchers (e.g., Stefansson et al., 2008) found three genetic deletions located on chromosomal regions 1q21.1, 15q11.2, and 15q13.3 that are associated with schizophrenia and psychosis. A genome wide survey of rare CNVs in a large sample of patients (n = 3,391) and controls (n = 3,181) discovered deletions of 12p11.23 and 16p12.1–p12.2 in some patients. However, further studies are needed to replicate these findings. Furthermore, it is still unknown how often these gene alterations are inherited, how often they may lead to schizophrenia, and how often individuals who possess a genetic vulnerability for schizophrenia pass onto their offspring despite the fact that they have never been diagnosed with the illness.

Table 2.1 Etiological Factors of Schizophrenia

Risk Genes
Neuregulin, Dysbindin, D-amino acid oxidase, Catechol-O-methyltransferase, Proline dehydrogenase, Reelin, serotonin type 2a receptor, dopamine D3 receptor
Early Insults: Prenatal, Perinatal, and Postnatal Risks
Viral Infections: herpes simplex, influenza, rubella
Toxins: Lead, alpha-aminolevulinic acid
Obstetric complications: Mother hypertention, loss of husband while being pregnant, malnutrition, delivery complications
Other Environmental Factors
Vitamin D deficiency, winter birth, high latitude, inner city residence, drug use, natural disasters
Brain Abnormality
Reduction in whole brain and hippocampal volume, low volume of total cortical gray matter, high volumes of white matter, ventricular, and basal ganglia; larger superior temporal gyri relative to brain size; lack of normal right-greater-than left hippocampal asymmetry; larger ventricles, smaller temporal lobes, reduced metabolism in frontal lobe, significant reduction of mid sagittal thalamus

Despite encouraging findings linking risk genes to schizophrenia, molecular genetic studies also reveal that there is significant overlap in the genes that contribute to schizophrenia and other psychiatric disorders like schizoaffective disorder, and the manic syndromes associated with Type 1 Bipolar Disorder, which also present psychotic symptoms (Cardno, Rijsdijk, Sham, Murray, & McGuffin, 2002; Potash, Willour, Chiu, Simpson, & Mackinnon, 2001). This indicates that "there are genetic vulnerabilities to psychosis in general, and that the expression of these vulnerabilities can take the form of schizophrenia or an affective psychosis, depending on other inherited and acquired risk factors" (Walker et al., 2004, p. 409).

Concluding Comments Regarding the Role of Genetics

The available data suggest that multiple genetic factors account many cases of schizophrenia (Nicolson et al., 2003). The genetic explanations of schizophrenia either take the additive format or interactive format, with the former indicating that a certain number of factors/genes work together to reach a critical threshold for schizophrenia to develop and the latter as multiple predisposing genes interacting with each other to cause schizophrenia (e.g., Tsuang, Stone, & Faraone, 2001). However, still yet to be identified are potential environmental and biological risk factors that may interact with genetic predispositions and lead to symptoms characteristic of schizophrenia.

Environment

As indicated in the previous section, the etiology of schizophrenia appears to involve genetic factors. Nevertheless, about 60% of all individuals with schizophrenia do not have a first or second degree relative with this disorder or known as having the illness. Further, the degree of concordance for schizophrenia among identical twins is only about 50%, indicating that risk factors in the environment may play a role in the development of schizophrenia. In fact, Tsuang et al. (2001) found that the nonshared environment of twins accounted for almost all of the liability for schizophrenia. Identified environmental factors that put an individual at risk of developing severe mental illnesses like schizophrenia include prenatal, perinatal, and postnatal factors and social stresses like trauma and stigma.

Prenatal Risks

Over the last two decades, researchers have theorized that toxic exposures and infections during prenatal phase may elevate the risk of later developing schizophrenia. For example, a growing body of literature supports the hypothesis that lead exposure that damages or disrupts the developing central nervous system is associated with schizophrenia. Opler et al. (2008) reported that elevated prenatal levels of alpha-aminolevulinic acid (alpha-ALA), a proxy for prenatal lead exposure (Pb), is associated with almost a twofold increase in risk for schizophrenia spectrum disorders later in life. Further, there was a 10–20-fold risk of developing schizophrenia following prenatal exposure to rubella (Brown, 2006; Brown et al., 2004; Brown et al., 2001). In addition, prenatal virus exposure in genetically high-risk individuals may increase the likelihood of an individual's developing schizophrenia. In addition, in a study examining the interaction between gene and environment, Carter found that 21% of schizophrenia candidate genes interact with influenza virus, 22% with herpes simplex virus1, and 13% with rubella. However, conclusive evidence of an in utero infectious etiology of schizophrenia remains elusive (Lewis & Levitt, 2002).

Research findings also suggest people who develop schizophrenia are more likely to be born in the winter and early spring or in higher latitudes when compared with the general population (Kinney et al., 2009; Torrey, Miller, Rawings, & Yolken, 1997). Two hypotheses have been put forth to explain these observations. One is associated with increased influenza infection of pregnant mothers in cold temperature and the other is related to possible Vitamin D deficiency due to lengthened time indoors and shortened exposure to sunlight in cold weather. Both prenatal exposure to influenza and Vitamin D deficiency have been found to be associated with the development of schizophrenia (McGrath, 1999; Torrey et al., 1997). However, people with other psychiatric illnesses like depression and bipolar were also likely born in winter (Lewis & Levitt, 2002). Therefore, more research is warranted to delineate factors that may contribute more to the development of schizophrenia.

Perinatal Risks

Several perinatal factors have been identified to be associated with increased risk for schizophrenia. General nutritional deprivation and lack of specific micronutrients during pregnancy have been implicated as risk factors for schizophrenia (Opler & Susser, 2005). Susser et al. (1996) found that the rates of schizophrenia almost doubled for individuals conceived under conditions of nutrient deprivation during early gestation. Body mass index or low birth weight is also found to be associated with schizophrenia. Low maternal BMI was significantly associated with schizophrenia in the adult offspring. This finding was independent of maternal age, race, education, or cigarette smoking during pregnancy.

In addition, Sørensen and colleagues proposed that maternal hypertension during pregnancy and its treatment with diuretics in the third trimester of pregnancy were independently related to the development of schizophrenia in the offspring, and the association remained significant after controlling from maternal diagnosis of schizophrenia (Sørensen, Mortensen, Reinisch, & Mednick, 2003). There was also a sevenfold risk of developing schizophrenia following exposure to influenza in the first trimester (Brown, 2008).

A meta-analysis of the effect of exposure to obstetric complications on the development of schizophrenia shows that those with obstetric complications are twice as likely to develop schizophrenia (Geddes & Lawrie, 1995). Obstetric complications refer to a broad class of negative events and child development during pregnancy, labor-delivery, and early neonatal period (McNeil, 1988). Furthermore, labor-delivery complications (LDCs) were associated with an increased risk of EOS (Verdoux et al., 1997). Those who developed schizophrenia by age 22 were 2.7 times more likely to have abnormal presentation at birth and 10 times more likely to have a complicated Caesarean section. In twin studies, LDCs, rather than negative pregnancy events, identify monozygotic twins of which one or both developed schizophrenia, but not twins who were not affected. Specifically, in instances where one twin has schizophrenia and the other does not and when one twin was affected with schizophrenia and was born second, there were high rates of prolonged labor and lower rates of complications during pregnancy. Nevertheless, if the twin affected with schizophrenia was born first, the rate of prolonged labor was low and the rate of complications during pregnancy was high (Verdoux et al.). However, it should be noted that 97% of those with labor-delivery complications in population-based studies do not develop schizophrenia, which indicates that LDCs have low predictive value for the appearance of schizophrenia (Lewis & Levitt, 2002). Based on the gene and environment interaction model, "the offspring born with LDCs of individuals with schizophrenia may be more likely to develop schizophrenia than the offspring born without LDCs, whereas the same degree of LDCs does not increase risk of schizophrenia in the offspring of control subjects" (Lewis & Levitt, p. 416).

Postnatal Risks

Among the few studies examining the relationship between infection during childhood and the risk of subsequent schizophrenia, Dalman et al. (2008), in their cohort study of more than one million Swedish participants, found a weak association between viral central nerve system infections during childhood and the later development of schizophrenia spectrum disorders. Among the different viral infections, only mumps and cytomegalovirus infections were found to be associated with increased risk for psychosis.

Trauma

Trauma is another environmental factor that may operate independently or interact with genetic vulnerability to trigger psychotic symptoms of schizophrenia (Morgan & Fisher, 2007). For instance, research findings indicate 35% of patients diagnosed as schizophrenia as adults had been removed from home due to neglect, doubling the rate of other psychiatric diagnosis (e.g., Robins, 1996). In the study of over 100 children with schizophrenia spectrum disorders, "13% had a history of physical abuse, 10% sexual abuse, 14% neglect, and 20% witnessed trauma in the past" (Frazier et al., 2007, p. 982).

Read and colleagues indicate that "child abuse is a causal factor for psychosis and 'schizophrenia' and, more specifically for hallucination, particularly voices commenting and command hallucinations" (Read, van Os, Morrison, & Ross, 2005, p. 330). Child abuse is also related to early age of onset and more positive symptoms. In the Finnish Adoptive Family Study of Schizophrenia, the risk elevated significantly if the adoptees were raised in families with unfavorable atmosphere, while the risk of schizophrenia of those with genetic vulnerability did not differ from those adoptees with no genetic risks if they were raised in families with a favorable atmosphere (Tienari et al., 1994). These findings support the role of negative life events in the development of schizophrenia.

Several models are used to explain the association between trauma and the development of schizophrenia (Read et al., 2005; Walker & Diforio, 1997). First, early traumatic experiences may predispose persons to be more psychologically and cognitively sensitive to emotional distress which may trigger psychotic symptoms. Specifically, negative beliefs about self (helpless, vulnerable), world, and others (dangerous, suspicious) are found to be associated with psychosis (e.g., Morrison, 2001), and so are positive beliefs about psychotic experiences (such as paranoid as a survival strategy). According to Read et al. (2005), the second model implicates faulty source monitoring. Hallucinations are strongly related to childhood abuse and they are often, however, memories of the traumatic experience indicative of PTSD rather than psychotic symptoms of schizophrenia. However, when individuals with abuse history confuse between inner experience (memory of the past) and outer experience (external event happening in the present) and when they contribute such internal event to an external event (which is called faculty source monitoring), they start to experience heightened level of distress and develop delusional explanations of the experience. Henquet, Krabbendam, Dautzenberg, Jolles, and Merckelback (2005) proposed that source monitoring difficulties are a "prominent feature of schizophrenia" (p. 57). Furthermore, faulty source monitoring is more related to visual, tactile, and olfactory hallucinations than to auditory ones. Third, Walker and Diforio (1997) proposed a traumagenic neurodevelopmental (TN) model in understanding the relationship between trauma and the development of schizophrenia. This TN model integrates social, psychological, and biological factors, and it proposes that one's brain is affected by environment throughout his or her life. They reported neurological abnormalities evidenced in schizophrenia patients in the brains of traumatized children. Such abnormalities include hippocampal damage, cerebral atrophy (loss of brain cells), ventricular enlargement, and reversed cerebral asymmetry, which were related to cognitive deficits such as memory and attention. Lastly, Walker and Diforio proposed the model of stress cascade and psychosis in schizophrenia that life stressors may trigger or exacerbate psychotic symptoms as they increase dopamine activity, particularly in the subcortical region of the limbic circuitry. It is important to note that not all individuals who have been diagnosed with schizophrenia have experienced trauma, thus, implicating other etiological influences.

Stigma

Stigma, as a structural discrimination and social adversity, not only starts after a person is diagnosed as schizophrenia, but may serve as a causal factor of schizophrenia in response to the behavioral expression of genetic risk. van Zelst (2009) hypothesized that individuals at the prodromal stage may manifest early signs of psychosis, such as paranoid reactions or odd speech. These behaviors may lead to negative social interactions and stigma which increase the risk of these individuals' transitioning to psychotic disorder in general and schizophrenia in particular.

Concluding Comments Regarding the Role of the Environment

Different environmental factors may play a role in the development of schizophrenia. However, currently, there is little evidence supporting any one environmental factor as playing a primary role in the development of schizophrenia. In many cases, it appears that environmental factors interact with genetic vulnerability to influence the development of schizophrenia.

Neurobiology

No single pathology has been found to account for all the cases of schizophrenia, including EOS, rather, several different etiological models have been proposed. The following addresses neurobiological basis of schizophrenia.

Brain Structure

Lab studies show abnormal brain structures among individuals of EOS (e.g., Lawrie, McIntosh, Hall, Owens, & Johnstone, 2008). Brain structural studies show that superior parietal lobe pathology, particularly on the right, was progressively more pronounced in COS cases. Positive association between age of onset of psychosis and right parietal gray matter volume in EOS were also reported. Parietal cortices regulate spatial representation and motor planning and goal directed attention set shifting. Deficits in these regions may be related to motor abnormalities, and they are more prominent in EOS (Burke, Androutsos, Jogia, Byrne, & Frangou, 2008).

In addition, the longitudinal assessment of EOS cases from the NIMH cohort found gray matter loss that appeared first in parietal regions and then spread to the prefrontal cortex (Vidal et al., 2006). Burke et al. (2008) investigated the effect of age of onset on front-parietal gray matter among adolescents with schizophrenia and found the earlier the onset of schizophrenia the less the gray matter volume in the right parietal lobe, and the longer the duration of the illness. The parietal cortices are associated with such cognitive functions as spatial representation, coordination, self monitored motor function, motor imagery, abstract motor planning, and goal directed attention shifting. Parietal abnormalities may also be associated with the inability to differentiate between self-produced and externally generated behavior, which is the hallmark of psychosis. Wood et al. (2003) postulate that reduced gray matter density may be responsible for cognitive impairments in spatial working memory and rapid information processing (tasks like story recall). In fact they suggest that the prefrontal cortex seems the most promising region in terms of prediction of later psychosis.

Furthermore, increased gray matter loss in EOS could be genetically influenced and a trait marker of individuals with EOS. Gogtay et al. (2003) found using NIMH COS data that significant gray matter reduction in younger healthy full siblings of COS in left prefrontal and bilateral temporal cortices relative to healthy controls. However, such cortical deficits in siblings disappeared by age 20, which suggests a "plastic or restitutive brain response in these nonpsychotic, nonspectrum siblings" (Gogtay, 2008, p. 33). Yoshihara et al. (2008) also found in a study of patients with EOS that the positive symptom score of Positive and Negative Symptom Scale (PANSS) (higher values indicating more severe symptom) is negatively correlated with gray matter volume in the right thalamus, and the positive symptom score of PANSS was positively related to cerebella white matter.

Several meta-analysis studies report bilateral reduced volume in hippocampus, indicative of potential markers of psychosis (Lawrie & Abukmeil, 1998; Wright et al., 2000). Structural imaging studies indicate that reductions in hippocampal volume occur during the transition from the premorbid to prodromal to the overtly psychotic phases of the illness (Matsumoto et al., 2001). However, the smaller hippocampal volume may not predict later psychosis but instead be a result of environmental insults such as obstetric complications.

Other brain regions have been examined as potential markers of later showing positive symptoms. Enlarged lateral ventricles were the first and most consistently reported brain abnormality in schizophrenia research. Sowell et al. (2000) also found symmetry ventricles in participants with EOS, whereas a larger ventricle in the left hemisphere was found in control participants. "It is probable that neuroanatomical cerebral abnormalities present prior to disease onset play an etiopathogenic role in the development of schizophrenia" (Mehler & Warnke, 2002).

Brain Chemistry

Researchers in the field of schizophrenia have been exploring neurochemistry bases for schizophrenia. Over the past four decades, dopamine and dopaminergic mechanisms have been a central hypothesis of the development of schizophrenia and the findings over the years have been reframing the theoretical explanations of such neural circuitry models of schizophrenia (Howes & Kapur, 2009). The dopamine hypothesis started in 1970s when it was believed that psychosis was caused by excessive transmission at dopamine receptor and antipsychotic drugs were invented to block these receptors to treat psychosis. However, this hypothesis did not delineate the relationship between the role of dopamine receptor and positive and negative symptoms, nor did it specify the link between genetics and neurodevelopmental deficits and specify the abnormal brain regions.

Latest findings from the past decade have modified the domapine hypothesis. Many recent findings link dopamine hyperfunction most closely to psychosis (positive symptoms), a hallmark of schizophrenia (Howes & Kapur, 2009). The latest dopamine hypothesis was enriched with findings from gene variants and environment risk factors that influence dopaminergic functions. Two major components of the current dopamine hypothesis are: (a) multiple hits – different gene variants, neural transmitters such as serotonin, norepinephrine, glutamate or y-aminobutyric acid (GABA), and environmental factors such as trauma and prenatal, perinatal, and postnatal factors, interact to result in dopamine dysfunction (Meyer & Feldon, 2009). (b) Dopamine regulation is linked to "psychosis" rather than schizophrenia. The exact diagnosis, therefore, "reflects the nature of the hits coupled with sociocultural factors and not the dopamine dysfunction per se" (Howes & Kapur, p. 555).

Concluding Comments Regarding the Role of Neurobiology

Neurobiological research findings indicate that the neuropathologies associated with schizophrenia are related to abnormalities in different localities of the brain. These abnormalities involve different brain structures, neurotransmitters, genetic variants, all of which may interact with environment factors to lead to symptoms associated with schizophrenia. Table 2.1 summarizes neurobiological findings of schizophrenia.

Concluding Comments

This chapter has presented the complicated etiology of schizophrenia in general and EOS in several sections. Despite the multitude of research exploring its causes, definitive causes of schizophrenia and EOS in particular remain elusive. As individuals with schizophrenia present a variety of symptoms at different stages of life under different circumstances, it is unlikely to find a single cause for schizophrenia, including EOS. This observation is consistent with the hypothesis that "schizophrenia is probably neither a single disease entity and nor is it a circumscribed syndrome – it is likely to be a conglomeration of phenotypically similar disease entities and syndromes" (Tandon, Nasrallah, & Keshavan, 2009, p. 1). Researchers generally agree on a multifaceted etiological model of schizophrenia, including genetic, neurobiological, neuroanatomical mechanisms, and environmental factors. Future studies are needed to clarify and specify the nature of the complex interplay among the different factors and their unique contribution to the development of schizophrenia in general and EOS in particular.

Chapter 3
Prevalence, Incidence, and Associated Conditions

This chapter explores the prevalence and incidence of Early Onset Schizophrenia (EOS, onset of symptoms prior to age 18 years). Additionally, EOS's association with other conditions will be examined, with special attention given to issues associated with comorbidity. Typical adjustment and outcomes are also briefly summarized to further describe associated conditions.

Prevalence and Incidence

The "prevalence" of a condition typically refers to the total number of people who currently have the condition, whereas "incidence" commonly refers to the number of new cases during a given time period. Given the chronic nature of EOS (onset prior to age 18 years), the annual incidence is relatively low, however, the cumulative prevalence is much higher. The lifetime prevalence of EOS in the general population has been examined in multiple studies. It has been estimated that about one in 10,000 children will develop some form of schizophrenic disorder, with childhood-onset schizophrenia (COS, onset prior to age 12 years) occurring in roughly one out of every 40,000 children (Asarnow & Asarnow, 2003; Nicolson & Rapoport, 1999). The typical age of onset of schizophrenia is between 16- and 35-years-old (Asarnow, Thompson, & McGrath, 2004), thus, EOS is relatively rare. Although EOS is typically considered a rare phenomenon, this is to some extent a misconception. While it is uncommon for the illness to develop in childhood, it has been estimated that almost one-third of persons with schizophrenia first experience psychotic symptoms during adolescence (Findling & Schulz, 2005).

Mueser and McGurk (2004) estimated the lifetime prevalence of schizophrenia (the proportion of individuals in the population who have ever manifested the illness and who are alive on a given day) to be one in 100, thus, based on this estimate, there would be approximately 2.5 million people (including adults, adolescents, and children) in the United States living with the disorder. Previous results of the National Comorbidity Survey revealed the lifetime prevalence rates of narrowly (schizophrenia or schizophreniform disorder) and broadly (all nonaffective psychoses)

H. Li et al., *Identifying, Assessing, and Treating Early Onset Schizophrenia at School*, Developmental Psychopathology at School, DOI 10.1007/978-1-4419-6272-0_3,

defined psychosis as 0.2% and 0.7%, respectively (Kendler et al., 1996). Estimates from the World Health Organization place the annual incidence rate at 0.22 out of 1,000 (Bromet, Dew, & Eaton, 1995), and the DSM-IV (2000) estimated the rate from 0.2% to 2%. To examine the prevalence and incidence of schizophrenia, McGrath et al. (2004) provide a systematic review of 188 studies conducted in 46 countries, published between 1965 and 2002 (see Table 3.1). For those studies that reported on lifetime prevalence, the mean was four per 1,000. DSM-IV-TR (APA, 2000) states that the lifetime prevalence of schizophrenia is often reported to be five to 15 per 1,000. For those studies that reported on point prevalence of schizophrenia (the proportion of individuals who manifest the illness at a given point of time), the mean point prevalence was 4.6 per 1,000. While there is substantial variation across studies, largely depending on the type of prevalence estimate used, McGrath et al. (2004) found that generally the prevalence of schizophrenia ranges from four to seven per 1,000 persons. Given the paucity of epidemiological studies focused on EOS, the information presented below is based on epidemiological studies of adults, unless otherwise noted.

Gender. The available research findings vary regarding gender and age of onset. Research is inconsistent as related to gender differences; some studies have found the ratio to be 2:1 (males to females; Green, Padron-Gayol, Hardesty, & Bassiri, 1992) and others report ratios as large as 5:1 (Hafner, Hambrecht, Loffler, Munk-Jorgenson, & Reichler-Rossier, 1998). The systematic review by McGrath et al. (2004) indicates that the incidence of schizophrenia is higher in males than females. A symposium on childhood-onset schizophrenia conducted by the European Child and Adolescent Psychiatry Association (Eggers et al., 1999) reported that there were no gender differences in age of first psychiatric symptoms and no significant difference in age at first psychotic symptom. However, the prevalence rates were reported to be earlier in males than in females. Previous findings indicate that males (a) suffer a psychotic episode at an earlier age, (b) show greater evidence of cognitive impairment, (c) evidence more neurological abnormalities, and (d) are more likely to have a more severe course of illness (Murray, Jones, Susser, van Os, & Cannon, 2003).

Socioeconomic Status (SES). Although schizophrenia appears across SES levels, it has been found to be more frequent in populations with lower SES (Kirkbride, Barker et al., 2008; Kirkbride, Boydell et al., 2008; Munk-Jorgensen & Mortensen, 1992). There are multiple interpretations of this relationship, for instance, it may be that the stress of poverty is a risk factor for manifesting schizophrenic symptoms, alternatively, the lower SES status may be due to the disorder itself; for example, a person with schizophrenia would have a more difficult time keeping a job or securing a high paying job.

Urbanization. Numerous studies report that the rates of schizophrenia are increased in inner city areas of Western societies. For instance, an early study revealed that first admission rates of schizophrenia were particularly high in areas of inner city Chicago, and decreased rates toward the periphery of the city (Faris & Dunham, 1939). In examining the specific characteristics of neighborhoods where higher rates were documented, the authors suggested that social isolation and lack of cohesion may be associated with the increased rates of schizophrenia.

Table 3.1 Summary of Recent Studies Examining the Incidence of Schizophrenia around the World (Adapted from McGrath et al., 2004. With permission)

Study	Nation; Area; Urban – rural	Period of observation	Age range; adjustment	Incidence[a] per 100,000 (Min–Max)[b]
Mahy, Mallett, Leff, and Bhugra, 1999	Barbados; Entire nation; Mixed urban – rural	1995	18–54; Adjusted	P: 28.2 (P: 4.0–32.0)
Messias, Sampaio, Messias, and Kirkpartick, 2000	Brazil; Northeast region; Mixed urban – rural	1964–1994	All ages; NA	P: 47.2
Bland, 1977	Canada; Entire nation; Mixed urban – rural	1972	All ages; Adjusted	M: 29.0 (F: 26.0)
Bland and Orn, 1978	Canada; Alberta province; Mixed urban – rural	1963	15–59; NA	P: 11.7
Bland, 1984	Canada; Entire nation; Mixed urban – rural	1978	All ages; NA	NA (M: 31.0 F: 22.0)
Iacono and Beiser, 1992	Canada;Vancouver City; Mixed urban – rural	1982–1984	16–50; NA	M: 11.1 (M: 5.6–11.1 F: 1.7–4.1)
Nicole, Lesage, and Lalonde, 1992	Canada; Quebec City; Mixed urban – rural	1983–1987	NA; NA	P: 30.7 (P: 8.6–30.7) M: 12.6–30.7 F: 4.9–22.4
D'Arcy, Rawson, Lydick, and Epstein, 1993	Canada; Saskatchewan; Mixed urban – rural	1977–1990	NA; NA	NA (P: 10.0–43.0)
Ma, 1980	China; Laoshan County; Mixed urban – rural	1967–1976	All ages; NA	P: 10.0 (P: 6.5–11.6)
Chen, 1984	China; Sijiging commune; Mixed urban – rural	1975–1981	NA; Adjusted	P: 11.0 (P: 6.8–15.6)
Yucun et al., 1988	China; Haidian district; Rural	1974–1977	15 & above; NA	NA (P: 11.0)
Folnegovic, Folnegovic-Smalc, and Kulcar, 1990	Croatia; Entire nation; Mixed urban – rural	1965–1984	All ages; NA	NA (P: 21.0–29.0 M: 21.0–30.0 F: 20.0–28.0)
Nielsen, 1976	Denmark; Samso Island; Rural	1957–1971	15 & above; NA	NA (P: 0.0–20.0)
Nielsen and Nielsen, 1977[c]	Denmark; Samso Island; Rural	1975	All ages; NA	P: 222.6 (M: 326.8 F: 120.3)
Munk-Jorgensen, 1986[c]	Denmark; Aarhus city; Urban	1984	15 & above; NA	P: 3.9 (P: 3.0–3.9)

(continued)

Table 3.1 (continued)

Study	Nation; Area; Urban – rural	Period of observation	Age range; adjustment	Incidence[a] per 100,000 (Min–Max)[b]
Munk-Jorgensen, 1986	Denmark; Entire nation; Mixed urban – rural	1970–1984	15 & above; Adjusted	NA(M: 7.5–12.5 F: 4.0–7.6)
Jablensky et al., 1992	Denmark; Aarhus city; Urban	1978–1979	15–54; Adjusted	NA (P: 9.0–16.0 M: 9.0–18.0 F: 5.0–13.0)
Munk-Jorgensen, Lutzhoft, Jensen, and Stromgren, 1992	Denmark; Entire nation; Mixed urban – rural	1971–1987	15 & above; NA	NA (M: 4.5–10.2 F: 1.5–5.1)
Munk-Jorgensen et al., 1992	Denmark; Entire nation; Mixed urban – rural	1971–1991	15 & above; NA	NA (M: 4.5–10.2 F: 1.9–5.1)
Mors and Sorensen, 1993	Denmark; Aarhus county; Mixed urban – rural	1969	18–49; NA	P: 11.0
Lynge and Jacobsen, 1995	Denmark; Entire Greenland; Mixed urban – rural	1980–1983	15–54; NA	NA (M: 41.0 F: 23.0)
Lyng, Mortensen, and Munk-Jorgensen, 1999	Denmark; Entire Greenland; Mixed urban – rural	1975	15 & above; NA	NA (M: 11.5–24.5 F: 3.6–7.4)
Schelin, 2000	Denmark; Copenhagen, other urban, & provincial towns; Mixed urban – rural	1978–1982	All ages; Adjusted	M: 8.6 (M: 8.6–26.1 F: 5.4–17.9)
Niskanen and Achte, 1972	Finland; Helsinki city; Urban	1950–1965	15 & above; NA	NA (P: 43.0–85.0)
Salokangas, 1979	Finland; Turku city; Urban	1949–1970	15 & above; NA	P: 39.9 (P: 29.9–49.1 M: 29.1–43.8 F: 42.8–53.1)
Kuusi, 1986	Finland; Helsinki city; Urban	1975	15–44; NA	P: 18.9 (M: NA F: NA)
Salokangas, 1993	Finland; Six health districts; Mixed urban – rural	1983–1984	All ages, 15–44; NA	NA (P: 12.0–30.0 M: 13.0–30.0 F: 12.0–29.0)
Lehtinen et al., 1996	Finland; South & North Finland; Mixed urban – rural	1970–1986	15–64; NA	48.5 (P: 25.3–90.0)
van Os, Galdos, Lewis, Bourgeois, and Mann 1993	France; Entire nation; Mixed urban – rural	1974–1978	All ages; Adjusted	NA (M: 11.8–15.1 F: 7.5–8.7)

(continued)

Table 3.1 (continued)

Study	Nation; Area; Urban – rural	Period of observation	Age range; adjustment	Incidence[a] per 100,000 (Min–Max)[b]
Hafner and An der Heiden, 1986 [75]	Germany; Mannheim city; Urban	1974–1980	15 & above; NA	P: 67.0 (P: 48.0–67.0)
Loffler and Hafner, 1999	Germany; Mannheim & Heidelberg cities; Urban	1987–1989	NA; Crude & adjusted	P: 9.5 (P: 9.5–27.7 M: NA F: NA)
Helgason, 1977	Iceland; Entire nation; Mixed urban – rural	1967	All ages; NA	P: 27.0
Jablensky et al., 1992	India; Chandigarh; Urban & rural	1978–1979	15–54; NA	NA (P: 9.0–44.0 M: 8.0–41.0 F: 9.0–48.0)
Rajkumar, Padmavati, Thara, and Sarada Menon, 1993	India; Madras: urban slum Urban	1988	15 & above; NA	P: 35.0
Walsh, 1992	Ireland; Entire nation; Mixed urban – rural	1974–1987	NA; NA	NA (P: 4.3–8.6)
Walsh, 1969	Ireland; Dublin city; Urban	1962	10 & above; Adjusted	P: NA (M: 57.0 F: 46.0)
O'Hare and Walsh, 1974	Ireland; Entire nation; NA	1965–1969	NA; NA	NA M: 60.0 (F: 44.0)
Ni Nuallain et al., 1984	Ireland Three counties: Carlow/ South Kildare, Westmeath & Roscommon; NA	1974–1977	15–64; NA	NA (M: 32.9 F:22.6)
Jablensky et al., 1992	Ireland; Dublin city; Urban	1978–1979	15–54; NA	NA (P: 9.0–22.0 M: 10.0–23.0 F: 8.0–21.0)
Repetto et al., 1988	Italy; Lombardy region; Mixed urban – rural	1981–1982	All ages, 15 & above, 10 & above; NA	P: 27.0 (P: 27.0–33.0 M: 26.0–32.0 F: 27.0–34.0)
Tansella, Balestrieri, Meneghelli, and Micciolo, 1991	Italy; South Verona city; Urban	1979–1988	14 & above; NA	NA (P: 9.9 M: 11.3 F: 8.5)

(continued)

Table 3.1 (continued)

Study	Nation; Area; Urban – rural	Period of observation	Age range; adjustment	Incidence[a] per 100,000 (Min–Max)[b]
De Salvia, Barbato, Salvo, and Zadro, 1993	Italy; Veneto region: Portogruaro health district; Mixed urban – rural	1982–1989	15 & above; NA	NA (P: 7.0–27.0 M: 17.0 F: 17.0)
Mata, Beperet, Madoz, and Psicost, 2000	Italy; Navarra region; Mixed urban – rural	1993–1997	15–54; NA	NA (P: 22.0)
Preti and Miotto, 2000	Italy; Entire nation; Mixed urban – rural	1984–1994	NA; NA	P: 8.8 (P: 5.3–8.8)
Hickling and Rodgers-Johnson, 1995	Jamaica; Entire nation; Mixed urban – rural	1992	15–54; Crude & adjusted	P: 21.6 (P: 11.6–23.6 M: 30.4 F: 16.6)
Jablensky et al., 1992	Japan; Nagasaki city; Urban	1978–1979	15–54; NA	NA (P: 10.0–20.0 M: 11.0–23.0 F: 9.0–18.0)
Ohta, Nakane, Nishihara, and Takemoto, 1992	Japan; Nagasaki city; Urban	1979–1980	15–54; NA	P: 21.0 (M: 25.0 F: 18.0)
Giel et al., 1980	The Netherlands; Groningen & Drenthe; Mixed urban – rural	1978–1979	15–44; NA	P: 2.9 (M: 2.8 F: 2.9)
Oldehinkel and Giel, 1995	The Netherland; Groningen city; Urban	1976–1990	15 & above; NA	NA (P: 6.3–14.0)
Peen and Dekker, 1997	The Netherlands; Hague areas; Mixed urban – rural	1991	15 & above; NA	P: 10.2 (M: NA F: NA)
van Os, Driessen, Gunther, and Delespaul, 2000	The Netherlands; Maastricht city; Urban	1986–1997	15–64; NA	P: 22.3
Selten 2001*	The Netherlands; Hague city; Urban	1997–1999	15–54; Adjusted	P: 2.1
Joyce, 1987	New Zealand; Entire nation; Mixed urban – rural	1974–1984	All ages; NA	P: 18.0 (P: 9.5–18.0)
Johannessen, 1985[c]	Norway; Rogaland county; Mixed urban – rural	1982–1983	All ages; NA	P: 2.8
Grawe, Levander, and Krueger 1991	Norway; Sor-Trondelag county; Mixed urban – rural	1986–1988	0–45; NA	P: 7.9

(continued)

Table 3.1 (continued)

Study	Nation; Area; Urban – rural	Period of observation	Age range; adjustment	Incidence[a] per 100,000 (Min–Max)[b]
Chowdhury, 1966[c]	Pakistan; East Pakistan; Mixed urban – rural	1961	All ages; NA	P: 0.4
Lieberman, 1974	Russia; Moscow city; Urban	1965–1969	NA; NA	NA (P: 19.1 M: 19.8 F: 18.5)
Rotshtein, 1982	Russia; Moscow city; Urban	1970–1976	All ages; NA	NA (P: 1.7 M: 1.8 F: 1.6)
Vul 1982	Russia; Siberia: Tumen, Nobolaska, Nizenvartosk, & Neffjugask cities; Mixed urban – rural	1984–1985	All ages; NA	NA (P: 5.0–27.0)
Jablensky et al., 1992	Russia; Moscow city; Urban	1978–1979	15–54; NA	NA (P: 12.0–28.0 M: 10.0–25.0 F: 14.0–31.0)
Tsoi and Chen, 1979	Singapore; Entire nation; Urban	1975	10 & above; NA	P: 29.3 (M: 33.7 F: 24.1)
Vazquez-Barquero et al., 1995	Spain; Cantabria region; Mixed urban – rural	1989–1990	All ages, & 15–54; NA	NA (P: 8.0–19.0 M: 8.4–18.8 F: 8.0–19.3)
Ösby et al., 2001	Sweden; Stockholm county; Mixed urban – rural	1978–1994	15–69; Adjusted	NA (M: 20.0–34.5 F: 15.0–33.0)
Svedberg 2001	Sweden; Stocholm: Three catchment areas; Urban	1991–1992	All ages, & 18–45; NA	P: 9.4 (P: 7.9–25.2)
Zolkowska et al., 2001*	Sweden; Malmo city; Urban	1998	18–64; NA	P: 27.4
Neehall, 1991[c]	Trinidad; NorthWest Peninsula; Mixed urban – rural	1986	15 & above; NA	P: 48.9
Bhugra et al., 1996	Trinidad; Entire nation; Mixed urban – rural	NA	15–54; Adjusted	P: 21.5 (P: 5.6–21.5)

(continued)

Table 3.1 (continued)

Study	Nation; Area; Urban – rural	Period of observation	Age range; adjustment	Incidence[a] per 100,000 (Min–Max)[b]
Adelstein, Downhan, Stein, and Susser, 1968	United Kingdom; Salford city; Urban	1959–1963	15 & above; NA	NA (M: 35.0 F: 26.0)
Mezey and Evans, 1971	United Kingdom; London: Edmonton; Urban	1963–1964	All ages; NA	NA (P: 280.0 M: 245.0 F: 313.0)
Eagles and Whalley, 1985	United Kingdom; Scotland: entire nation; Mixed urban – rural	1969–1978	NA; Adjusted	NA (P: 11.8–19.6)
Giggs 1986	United Kingdom; Nottingham city; Urban	1975–1979	15–59; NA	P: 30.5
Al Mousawi and Dunstan, 1998	United Kingdom; Scotland: entire nation; Mixed urban – rural	1963–1991	15–64; NA	NA (M: 11.4–23.7 F: 6.3–27.3)
Eagles, Hunter, and McCance, 1988	United Kingdom; Scotland: Grampian, Orkney & Shetland; Mixed urban – rural	1969–1984	NA; Adjusted	NA (P: 6.0–17.9)
De Alarcon and Seagroatt, 1990	United Kingdom; Oxfordshire; Mixed urban – rural	1975–1986	15 & above; Adjusted	NA (M: 19.0–33.0 F: 13.0–27.0)
Der, Gupta, and Murray, 1990	United Kingdom; England & Wales; Mixed urban – rural	1950–1986	NA; NA	NA (M: 9.0–18.0 F: 8.0–16.0)
Prince and Phelan, 1990	United Kingdom; England & Wales; Mixed urban – rural	1970–1985	NA; NA	NA (P: 8.0–16.0)
Bamrah, Freeman, Goldberg, 1991	United Kingdom; Salford city; Urban	1974–1984	All ages, &15 & above; NA	P: 28.0 (P: 7.0–28.0)
Harrison, Cooper, and Gancarczyk, 1991	United Kingdom; Nottingham city; Urban	1975–1987	15–64; NA	NA (P: 9.8–15.5)
Ring et al., 1991	United Kingdom; Manchester city; Urban	NA	16–49; Adjusted	NA (M: 19.0 F: 14.0)

(continued)

Table 3.1 (continued)

Study	Nation; Area; Urban – rural	Period of observation	Age range; adjustment	Incidence[a] per 100,000 (Min–Max)[b]
Jablensky et al., 1992	United Kingdom; Nottingham city; Urban	1978–1979	15–54; NA	NA (P: 14.0–22.0)
Geddes, Black, Whalley, and Eagles, 1993	United Kingdom; Scotland: entire nation; Mixed urban – rural	1969–1988	All ages; Adjusted	NA (M: 7.4–14.7 F: 4.8–11.7)
Castle and Murray, 1993	United Kingdom; Camberwell city; Urban	1965–1984	All ages, <45, >45; Adjusted	NA (M: 9.0–14.8 F: 6.0–17.6)
Kendell, Malcolm, and Adams, 1993	United Kingdom; Scotland: Edinburgh city; Urban	1971–1989	19 & above; Adjusted	NA (P: 11.0–21.5)
van Os et al., 1993	United Kingdom; Entire nation; Mixed urban – rural	1973–1979	All ages; Adjusted	NA (M: 8.8–15.1 F: 7.5–12.1)
Goldacre, Shiwach, and Yeates, 1994	United Kingdom; Oxfordshire; Mixed urban – rural	1975	0–64; NA	M: 8.7 (F: 5.6)
Prince and Phelan, 1994	United Kingdom; Camberwell & Gloucester; Urban	NA	NA; NA	NA (P: 12.0–26.0)
van Os, Castle, Takei, Der, and Murray, 1996*	United Kingdom; Camberwell; Urban	1988–1992	16 & above; Adjusted	P: 15.3
McNaught et al., 1997	United Kingdom; London: Hampstead area; Urban	1986–1991	All ages, 15–54, & 15 & above; NA	NA (P: 10.0–21.0)
Cavanagh and Shajahan, 1999	United Kingdom; Scotland: entire nation; Mixed urban – rural	1980–1995	All ages; NA	NA (M: 11.5–16.0 F: 6.0–13.0)
Boydell et al., 2001	United Kingdom; London: Camberwell Mixed urban – rural	1988–1997	16 & above Adjusted	NA (P: 3.0–38.0)
Dunham, 1965	USA; Detroit: Cass & Conner-Burbank; Urban	1958	15 & above; NA	P: 124.0 (P: 45.0–330.0)

(continued)

Study	Nation; Area; Urban – rural	Period of observation	Age range; adjustment	Incidence[a] per 100,000 (Min–Max)[b]
Eaton, 1974	USA; Maryland state; Mixed urban – rural	1965	All ages; NA	P: 30.0 (P: 23.0–60.0)
Jablensky et al., 1992	USA; Honolulu city; Urban	1978–1979	15–54; NA	NA (P: 9.0–16.0 M: 10.0–18.0 F: 8.0 14.0)
Tien and Eaton, 1992	USA; New Haven, Baltimore, St Louis, Durham, Los Angeles; Urban	1980–1984	18 & above; Adjusted	P: 200.0 (P: 40.0–710.0)

[a]Rates for *persons (P), males(M) & females(F)* . First row: rates associated with the reported numerator but not necessarily with the denominator; NA indicates no associated rate for any numerator

[b]Where multiple rates available, the minimum and maximum rates shown in brackets

[c]Rates are calculated

[*]Rates for migrant groups also available (rate details in Table 3.2)

NA = Not available

Full manuscript available online at http://www.biomedcentral.com/1741-7015/2/13

Full table available online at http://www.biomedcentral.com/imedia/1144262997341774/sup4.doc

Studies in Northern Europe have also reported an increased rate of schizophrenia associated with larger cities, relative to more rural areas (e.g., Lewis, David, Andreasson, & Alleback, 1992; Marcelis et al., 1998; Mortensen et al., 1999; Peen & Dekker, 1997). A "social drift" hypothesis has been profferred, suggesting that there is a tendency for persons with schizophrenia (present or incipient) to move into more urbanized or deprived areas. A variation is the "social residue" hypothesis, proposing that as a city develops, more able persons move out to suburbs, thus leaving a residual population with a higher risk of psychiatric disorders. Possible influences associated with urbanization include, social isolation, psychosocial stress, drug abuse, social class, obstetric complications, poor nutrition, and infectious diseases (Boydell & Murray, 2006).

Developmental Level. Schizophrenia with an earlier age of onset and a more chronic (as opposed to sudden) course is more likely to remain a persistent and recurrent psychological impairment. Therefore, adolescents diagnosed with schizophrenia tend to have a less favorable outcome than those diagnosed during adulthood and are more likely to suffer lingering symptoms or require residential care (Orr & Castle, 2003).

Ethnicity. Several studies suggest that certain ethnic minority groups may have an elevated incidence of schizophrenia (Eaton & Levav, 1982; Fearon et al., 2006; Kirkbride, Barker et al., 2008; Raman & Murphy, 1972). For instance, Keith, Reiger, and Rae (1991) found that schizophrenia is more prevalent in the African American population, although this may be confounded by previously reported findings revealing that socioeconomic status has been found to be associated with increased incidence. The *DSM-IV-TR* indicates that studies from the United Kingdom and the United States suggest that schizophrenia may be diagnosed more often in African Americans and Asian Americans than in other racial groups (APA, 2000). Other scholars have examined the influence of social capital to explore how societal stressors may influence increased rates among individuals within ethnic minority groups (Kirkbride, Boydell, et al., 2008); these findings may have implications related to increased rates among specific ethnic groups and migrants.

Migrant Status. Early research revealed an association between migrant status and increased risk of schizophrenia (Odegar, 1932). Contemporary scholarship has further supported this link, for instance, in the United Kingdom, rates have been shown to be higher among in both Afro-Caribbean migrants (Harrison, 1990) and other migrant groups (Aesop Study Team, 2002; Coid et al., 2008). Additional studies from Denmark (Cantor-Graae, Pedersen, McNeil, & Mortensen, 2000), the Netherlands (Selton et al., 2001), and Sweden (Zolkowska, Cantor-Graae, & McNeil, 2001) have also revealed an increased risk of schizophrenia among migrants. Moreover, the recent systematic review by McGrath et al. (2004) indicates an increased incidence among migrant groups relative to native-born individuals (summary of studies in Table 3.2). Explanations of this increased incidence among migrant groups are tentative but include the possibility of stressful life experiences impacting the onset of schizophrenia (Kirkbride, Barker et al., 2008; Kirkbride, Boydell et al., 2008).

Criminal and Violent Behaviors. Epidemiological evidence reveals that while the proportion of societal violence attributable to persons with schizophrenia is relatively small, this group of persons is significantly more likely to be violent than members of the general population. For instance, Volvavka et al. (1997) estimated that 20% of patients with schizophrenia had previously assaulted another person. It is notable that for more than half of these patients, the assault was reported to coincide with the onset of the illness. Studies also reveal a relatively high rate of assaults among inpatients with schizophrenia (Karson & Bigelow, 1987; Walker & Seifer, 1994). A study in Switzerland revealed that persons with schizophrenia were up to four times more likely to have been convicted of a violent offense (Spitzer et al., 1990). Another study of young adults revealed that a diagnosis of schizophreniform disorders more than doubled the risk of violence (Arseneault, Moffitt, Caspi, Taylor, & Silva, 2000). A study of homicide in Finland (Eronen, 1996) revealed that schizophrenia was associated with an increase in homicide for both men and women (eight and 6.5 times, respectively). Finally, a study in Australia indicated that relative to the general population, persons with schizophrenia were four times more likely to be convicted of interpersonal violence and ten times more likely to be convicted of homicide (Wallace et al., 1988). Overall, most researchers conclude that the association between schizophrenia and violence is significant even when demographic factors are considered (Walsh & Buchana, 2006). Substance abuse and acute psychotic symptoms have been found to discriminate those with schizophrenia who are at increased risk of committing violent acts (Rasanan et al., 1998; Swanson et al., 1990; Taylor & Gunn, 1984; Wallace et al., 1998).

Summary. The following provides a brief summary of epidemiological information considering studies regarding schizophrenia. EOS is relatively rare in the U.S. and internationally, with about one in 10,000 children developing some form of schizophrenic disorder. Most epidemiological studies focus on adults with schizophrenia, with limited research addressing EOS specifically. Findings regarding gender ratios are not consistent; some findings suggest that males (a) suffer a psychotic episode at an earlier age, (b) show greater evidence of cognitive impairment, (c) evidence more neurological abnormalities, and (d) are more likely to have a more severe course of illness. Rates of schizophrenia appear to be increased in inner city areas of western societies and within areas with low socio-economic status (e.g., low income). A few studies suggest that African American and Asian American populations may be diagnosed more frequently in the United States. Scholarship has also revealed an association between migrant status and increased risk of schizophrenia. Finally, research reveals that the proportion of societal violence attributable to persons with schizophrenia is relatively small, however, this group of persons is significantly more likely to be violent than members of the general population.

Associated Conditions

Psychosis can occur across a range of childhood disorders. For instance, when psychotic symptoms occur during manifestation of Major Depressive Disorder, Bipolar Disorder, Obsessive-Compulsive Disorder, or Posttraumatic Stress Disorder, the psychotic symptoms may be considered to be evidence of the severity of that condition, rather than an indicator of a separate disorder. There is significant evidence revealing that EOS is often comorbid (simultaneous occurrence of two or more conditions) with other *DSM-IV-TR* (APA, 2000) disorders. For instance, Russell, Bott, and Sammons (1989) reported that 68% of their sample of children (4–13 years) with schizophrenia met criteria for another *DSM-III* (APA, 1980) diagnosis. The most common codiagnoses were atypical depression or dysthymic disorder (37%) and Conduct Disorder or Oppositional Defiant Disorder (31%). A more recent study (McClellan, Breiger, McCurry, & Hlastala, 2003) reported similarly high rates of comorbidity among youth with schizophrenia (69%), as well as youth with psychosis NOS (not otherwise specified, 85%). As discussed in the *DSM-IV-TR*, disorganized speech is commonly observed in numerous disorders with childhood onset (e.g., Communication Disorder, Pervasive Developmental Disorders), as is disorganized behavior (e.g., Attention-deficit/Hyperactivity Disorder, Stereotypic Movement Disorder; APA, 2000). Thus, it is imperative that professionals should give due consideration to these more common childhood disorders. Given early controversies regarding the relationship between autism spectrum disorders and schizophrenia, it is notable that there does not appear to be an elevated risk of schizophrenia among samples of children with autism or other pervasive developmental disorders (Burd & Kerbeshian, 1987; Volkmar & Cohen, 1991). There is also the problem of early misdiagnosis. For instance, Werry,

Table 3.2 Summary of Recent Migrant studies Examining the Incidence of Schizophrenia around the World (Adapted from McGrath et al., 2004. With permission)

Study	Nation; Area; Urban – rural	Period of observation	Age range; Adjustment	Population groups	Incidence per 100,000 population: Male	Female	Persons
Krupinski and Cochrane, 1980	Australia; Victoria; Mixed urban – rural	1970–1972	15 & above; Crude & Adjusted	Native	91.0	99.0	–
				British	83.0	64.0	–
				German	165.0	176.0	–
				Italian	117.0	125.0	–
				Polish	216.0	388.0	–
Weyerer and Hafner, 1992	Germany; Mannheim; Urban	1974	NA; Adjusted	Native			
				Inner	–	–	168.0
				Intermediate	–	–	102.0
				Outer zone	–	–	78.0
				Foreign born:	–	–	
				Inner	–	–	108.0
				Intermediate	–	–	95.0
				Outer zone	–	–	98.0
Zolkowska et al., 2001[c] [33]	Sweden; Malmo city; Urban	1998	18–64; NA	Native			21.9
				Immigrants			44.5
				All groups			27.4

(continued)

Table 3.2 (continued)

Study	Nation; Area; Urban – rural	Period of observation	Age range; Adjustment	Population groups	Incidence per 100,000 population		
					Male	Female	Persons
Selten, 1994	The Netherlands; Entire nation; Mixed urban – rural	1986–1990	15 & above; NA	Native			
				1986	31.0	19.0	–
				1987	26.0	19.0	–
				1988	23.0	16.0	–
				1989	22.0	15.0	–
				1990	21.0	15.0	–
				Surinamese			
				1986	186.0	66.0	–
				1987	154.0	56.0	–
				1988	142.0	32.0	–
				1989	133.0	45.0	–
				1990	136.0	46.0	–
				Antillean			
				1986	256.0	61.0	–
				1987	187.0	45.0	–
				1988	161.0	59.0	–
				1989	127.0	58.0	–
				1990	112.0	32.0	–
				Turk			
				1986	14.0	11.0	–
				1987	18.0	7.0	–
				1988	22.0	6.0	–
				1989	26.0	15.0	–
				1990	22.0	7.0	–
				Moroccan			
				1986	79.0	8.0	–
				1987	87.0	18.0	–
				1988	90.0	13.0	–
				1989	77.0	21.0	–
				1990	66.0	16.0	

Selten[c,d]1997	The Netherlands;Entire nation;	1983–1992	15–59;Adjusted	Native			
	Mixed urban – rural			Broad	2.47	1.27	–
				Restricted	1.02	0.49	–
				Surinamese			
				Broad	9.26	3.67	–
				Restricted	5.43	1.81	–
				NT Antillean			
				Broad	9.79	4.02	–
				Restricted	5.59	1.71	–
Selten [c,d]2001	The Netherlands;	1997–1999	15–54;	First generation: 15–54 years	8.5	3.1	–
	Hague city;		Adjusted	Native	20.3	16.8	–
	Urban			Surinamese	38.2	0.0	–
				NT Antillean	10.1	0.0	–
				Turk	53.4	6.1	–
				Moroccan	3.9	7.6	–
				Other, Westernised	16.8	16.5	–
				Other (nonwestern)	18.6	4.9	–
				Second generation 15–29	66.1	66.9	–
				years	0.0	0.0	–
				Native	0.0	0.0	–
				Surinamese	142.2	44.8	–
				NT Antillean	32.5	6.6	–
				Turk			
				Moroccan	8.5	3.1	–
				Other	26.5	23.4	–
				First & second generation	31.8	0.0	–
				15–54 years	8.9	0.0	–
				Native	60.9	10.8	–
				Surinamese	13.2	11.0	–
				NT Antillean			–
				Turk			
				Moroccan			
				Other			

(continued)

Table 3.2 (continued)

Study	Nation; Area; Urban – rural	Period of observation	Age range; Adjustment	Population groups	Incidence per 100,000 population		
					Male	Female	Persons
Hemsi, 1967	United Kingdom; Camberwell & Lambeth; Urban	1961	NA;NA	Native	27.0	20.0	24.0
				West Indian	131.0	51.0	91.0
Giggs, 1973	United Kingdom; Nottingham; Urban	1963–1969	15–44 NA	Native	–	–	120.0
				Irish	–	–	709.0
				European	–	–	720.0
				Indian/Pakistani	–	–	740.0
				West Indian	–	–	790.0
Rwegellera, 1977[d]	United Kingdom; Camberwell; Urban	1965–1968	15 & above; Adjusted	Native	–	–	12.0
				West African, Std	590.0	151.0	105.0
				West Indian, Std	170.0	30.0	32.0
				West African	–	–	418.0
				West Indian	–	–	92.0
Carpenter and Brockington, 1980	United Kingdom; Manchester city; Urban	1973–1975	15–45; NA	Native	–	–	20.0
				Indian	–	–	120.0
				Afro-Caribbean	–	–	111.0
Hitch and Rack, 1980	United Kingdom; Bradford; Urban	1968–1970	16–64; NA	Native	27.0	30.0	–
				Foreign-born	102.0	145.0	–

Dean, Downing, and Shelley, 1981a	United Kingdom; Southeast England; Mixed urban – rural	1976	All ages; Adjusted	Native	9.6	9.9	–
				Indian	–	–	207.1
				Pakistani	–	–	77.1
				African	–	–	615.4
				West Indian	–	–	–
				All ethnic	–	–	281.4
Dean, Walsh, Downing, and Shelley, 1981b	United Kingdom; Southeast England; Mixed urban – rural	1976	All ages; Adjusted	Native	30.1	30.0	7.9
				Irish			–
Cochrane and Bal, 1987	United Kingdom; England & Wales; Mixed urban – rural	1981	16 & above; Adjusted	Native	12.0	12.0	–
				Irish	13.0	25.0	–
				Caribbean	43.0	33.0	–
				Indian	13.0	19.0	–
				Pakistani	19.0	12.0	–
McGovern and Cope, 1987	United Kingdom; Birmingham; Urban	1980–1983	M:16–64 F:16–59; NA	Native 30 years	9.8	13.3	–
				+Native 16–29 years	20.5	7.0	–
				Afro-Caribbean 30 years+	45.3	52.8	–
				Afro-Caribbean 16–29 years	138.0	98.0	
				General populationICD9			
				DSM3			
				Caribbean 30–34 years			
				ICD9			16.0
				DSM3	–	–	10.0
				Caribbean	–	–	197.0
Harrison, Owens, Holton, Neilson, and Boot, 1988[e]	United Kingdom; Nottingham; NA	1984–1986	16–44; NA	16–29 years	–	–	169.0
				ICD9	–	–	291.0
				DSM3	–	–	175.0

(continued)

Table 3.2 (continued)

Study	Nation; Area; Urban – rural	Period of observation	Age range; Adjustment	Population groups	Incidence per 100,000 population		
					Male	Female	Persons
Cochrane and Bal, 1989	United Kingdom; Entire nation; Mixed urban – rural	1981	16 & above; Adjusted	Native	9.0	9.0	–
				Scottish	10.0	15.0	–
				Welsh	10.0	11.0	–
				N Irish	18.0	17.0	–
				Irish	18.0	22.0	–
				Caribbean	39.0	35.0	–
				Indian	11.0	18.0	–
				Pakistani	19.0	12.0	–
				German	11.0	7.0	–
				Italian	16.0	13.0	–
				American	13.0	6.0	–
				Kenyan	19.0	6.0	–
				Polish	24.	34.0	–
				Cypriot	18.0	8.0	–
				Hong Kong (Chinese)	7.0	29.0	–
Castle, Wessely, Der, and Murray, 1991	United Kingdom; Camberwell; Urban	1965–1984[m]	NA;Adjusted	Native			
				1965–1969	–	–	8.8
				1970–1974	–	–	9.8
				1975–1979	–	–	6.0
				1980–1984	–	–	4.0
				West Indian			
				1965–1969	–	–	46.7
				1970–1974	–	–	79.9
				1975–1979	–	–	70.3
				1980–1984	–	–	50.8

Thomas et al., 1993	United Kingdom; Manchester; Urban	1984–1987	16 & above; NA	Native	–	–	35.0
				16–29 years	–	–	23.0
				30–34 years	–	–	1 .6
				45 years+	–	–	35.0
				Asian	–	–	73.0
				16–29 years	–	–	49.0
				30–34 years	–	–	320.0
				45 years+	–	–	0.0
				Afro-Caribbean			45.0
				16–29 years			
				30–34 years			
				45 years+			
King, Coker, Leavey, Hoare, and Johnson-Sabine, 1994	United Kingdom; London: Haringey; Urban	1991–1992	16–54Adjusted	Native	–	–	12.4
				Black	–	–	53.0
				Caribbean	–	–	41.0
				African	–	–	81.0
				Other	–	–	46.0
				Total	–	–	45.0
				Asian	–	–	153.0
				Indian	–	–	48.0
				Pakistani	–	–	60.0
				Other			22.0
				Total			
				Total (all groups)			
van Os et al., 1996	United Kingdom; Camberwell; Urban	1988–1992	16 & above;Adjusted	Native	–	–	7.8
				Afro-Caribbean African	–	–	34.4
				All	–	–	53.2
					–	–	15.3

(continued)

Table 3.2 (continued)

Study	Nation; Area; Urban – rural	Period of observation	Age range; Adjustment	Population groups	Incidence per 100,000 population Male	Female	Persons
Bhugra et al., 1997	United Kingdom; Ealing, and South Southwark & East Lambeth Urban	1991–1993	18–64; Adjusted	Native	41.9	19.1	30.0
				Asian	32.1	29.9	36.0
				Afro-Caribbean	95.8	28.3	59.0
Harrison et al., 1997[c]	United Kingdom; Nottingham; NA	1992–1994	16–64;Crude & Adjusted	General population[e]	–	–	6.0
				Afro-Caribbean			60.0
Goater et al., 1999	United Kingdom; London; Urban	1992	16–54;Adjusted	Native	–	–	12.0
				Black	–	–	46.0
				Asian	–	–	60.0
				Other			39.0
Malzberg, 1967	USA;New York; Mixed rural/urban	1960–1961	?;NA	New York born	–	–	29.9
				Internal migrants			61.6

[a]Used Rate Ratio (RR) wherever reported
[b]Native: reference population
[c]Rates calculated (rates calculated where both numerator and denominator were reported)
[d]Rates based on person-years of exposure (not presented); RRs were extracted from the study
[e]General population= Other than Afro-Caribbeans (used as a reference population)
Note: See Glossary (Appendix 1) for definitions of the key variables
Full manuscript available online at http://www.biomedcentral.com/1741-7015/2/13
Full table available online at http://www.biomedcentral.com/imedia/1144262997341774/sup4.doc

McClellan, and Chard (1991) reported that over half of the children (patients ages 7–17 years) in their study who had an eventual mood disorder were initially diagnosed with schizophrenia. In another study, following 209 youth initially diagnosed with schizophrenia before age 18 over 10 years, many youth were later reported to have personality disorders (Thomsen, 1996).

Learning Disability and Special Education. The point prevalence of schizophrenia among individuals with learning disabilities has been estimated at 3%, which is higher than the estimate of 1% within the general population (Doody, Johnstone, Sanderson, Owens, & Muir, 1998; Turner, 1989, Tyrer & Dunstan 1997). In examining childhood backgrounds of individuals with schizophrenia, Willinger, Heiden, Meszaros, Formann, and Aschauer (2001) found that individuals with schizophrenia more frequently presented learning disabilities, relative to their siblings. A recent study by Morgan, Leonard, and Jablensky (2008) found that 37–52% of those with intellectual disability had co-occurring schizophrenia. Moreover, Bouras et al. (2004) reported that individuals with intellectual disability and schizophrenia spectrum psychoses were more debilitated by the co-occurring disorder than those with the same disorder but without intellectual disability.

Diagnosis of EOS may be challenging among individuals with learning disabilities as a result of communication problems, both comprehension and expression. Research also reveals some qualitative differences in symptoms in comparing individuals with learning disabilities and others (Reid 1989; Turner, 1989), for instance, complex hallucinations and complex delusions are less common among individuals with learning disabilities. The onset of schizophrenia symptoms may be less noticeable among individuals with learning disabilities, as they are more likely to include a decline in functioning, deterioration of self-help skills, and social withdrawal, rather than hallucinations and delusions which may only become salient over time. It should also be noted, that there is one study that reported no differences between individuals with the dual diagnosis of learning disability and schizophrenia, compared to those with schizophrenia only (Meadows et al., 1991); however, this may be a result of the specific participants in the sample.

Among individuals with learning disabilities, it has been documented that there is often a long delay between the start of symptoms and the diagnosis (James, Mukherjee, & Smith, 1996). As a result of the negative impact of symptoms of EOS on academic performance, learning, and peer relationships, many children with schizophrenia receive special education services at school. Chapter 6 provides further discussion of important psychoeducational assessment considerations and information pertaining to special education.

Summary. Symptoms of schizophrenia and related classifications are also frequently manifested within other disorder classifications. For instance, psychosis is a frequent symptom across multiple mental health classifications (e.g., Depression, Bipolar Disorder, Obsessive-Compulsive Disorder, Posttraumatic stress Disorder), disorganized speech is commonly observed in numerous disorders with childhood onset (e.g., Communication Disorder, Pervasive Developmental Disorders), as is disorganized behavior (e.g., Attention-deficit/Hyperactivity Disorder, Stereotypic Movement Disorder). Children with pervasive developmental disorders (e.g., Autistic and

Asperger's Disorders) often have social difficulties and language impairments, thus, these developmental disorders can be confused with a diagnosis of schizophrenia. Moreover, comorbidity (or dual diagnosis) is common. The common symptoms and variation in early manifestation of behaviors may make it difficult for clinicians to distinguish these disorders from one another (Rowland, Lesesne, & Abramowitz, 2002). The controversy regarding symptom overlap, dual diagnosis, differential diagnosis, and comorbidity continues to propel debates regarding the value and meaning of the classification criteria delineated in the *DSM IV-TR*, with some scholars proposing alternative procedures for assessment and case formulation among children (Achenbach, 1998). Among individuals with learning disabilities, rates of schizophrenia are higher than within the general population (3% and 1%, respectively). As a result of communication problems, early identification is challenging and diagnosis of schizophrenia is frequently delayed. Youth with EOS are likely to receive special education support services.

Adjustment and Outcomes

To better understand associated conditions and premorbid behaviors, Alaghband-Rad et al. (1995) reviewed the premorbid histories of 23 children meeting *DSM-III-R* criteria for schizophrenia with onset before age 12 years and compared these with childhood data of later-onset schizophrenia patients. Findings revealed greater delay in language development, more premorbid speech and language disorders, learning disorders, and disruptive behavior disorders. Thus, Alaghband-Rad et al.(1995) concluded that EOS represents a more malignant form of the disorder. Similarly, Hollis (1995, 2003) revealed that premorbid social, motor, and language impairments are especially notable in EOS compared to other forms of psychiatric disorders with early onset.

There are relatively few longitudinal studies examining the long-term psychopathological and psychosocial outcomes of early-onset schizophrenia, thus, relatively little is known. The existing literature describes a more severe course of illness among persons with EOS, compared with adult-onset schizophrenia. The following provides a brief summary of relevant research findings.

Werry et al. (1991) investigated 59 former child and adolescent psychotic patients, only 17% were doing well (displaying healthy adjustment and adaptation) at follow-up (1–16 years later). The authors described EOS as a chronic or relapsing disorder. Gillberg, Hellgren, and Gillberg (1993) found disconcerting results in their follow-up study, with only 13% of the 23 former patients showed a good outcome 11–17 years after follow-up. Asarnow et al. (1994) assessed a sample of 18 patients diagnosed with EOS, finding a good level of psychosocial functioning in only 28% of the cases and 17% showed a deteriorating course. Another follow-up study by Maziade et al. (1996) also highlighted the deleterious course of EOS, in their sample of 40 patients, only 5% of patients achieved a total recovery after a mean follow-up interval of 14.8 years. In 34% of the cases, the outcome was described as poor, in 40% as very poor.

In a follow-up study 10 years after the first psychotic episode, Lay, Blanz, Hartmann, and Schmidt (2000) reexamined 65 individuals with EOS; serious social disability was found in 66% of patients. Fleishhaker et al. (2005) reassessed 81 youth with EOS 9.5 years after the onset of the disorder, a good outcome was found in 20% of the individuals and 42% had a very poor outcome or gross impairment. They also investigated psychosocial factors like education, living conditions, and occupational situation at follow-up, revealing that only 29% were employed on a nonsheltered basis and half of the patients lived in assisted-living establishments.

Schmidt et al. (1995) completed a follow-up study with 97 individuals with EOS (mean age of onset 16 years, mean follow-up interval 7.4 years). At follow-up, 30% of the patients were semi-dependent or dependent, 72% still required psychiatric treatment, 44% were at least moderately impaired with regard to educational, occupational functions, and 58% with regard to social functions. Comparison with schizophrenia beginning in adulthood showed that the impairment in social function was much greater in the younger group of patients. Further research is warranted to examine subgroups of individuals with EOS to better understand how individuals with the specific characteristics (e.g., paranoid, disorganized, catotonic) may adjust over time.

Findings from a recent retrospective study of individuals who were younger than 18-years-old and received their first inpatient treatment due to schizophrenia indicated that at follow-up (mean 13.5 years later), 22% reported having acute schizophrenic symptoms, 31% described symptoms of depression, 37% reported having tried to commit suicide or had considered seriously, and 78% were still in outpatient treatment (Reichert, Kreiker, Mehler-Wex, & Warnke, 2008). Compared to the general population, the number of patients who did not graduate from high school was relatively high (3% and 19%, respectively). As a consequence, educational problems led in many cases to occupational difficulties, with 19% working in the open market. In addition, 48% still lived with their parents and 33% lived in assisted or semi-assisted living conditions. In contrast, the literature suggests that adult onset schizophrenia is more likely to be associated with periods of improvement, a higher level of psychosocial functioning, and a better overall outcome. Chapter 7 discusses treatment strategies to facilitate the development, adjustment, and adaptation of individuals with EOS.

Summary. In addition to comorbidity of other mental health disorders, as discussed earlier in this chapter, associated conditions include greater delay in language development, more premorbid speech and language disorders, learning disorders, and disruptive behavior disorders. Educational and occupational difficulties are frequently reported among individuals with EOS. Follow-up findings reveal a poor course of outcomes associated with EOS. In comparison to follow-up studies of adult-onset schizophrenia, collectively, these results support the assertion that psychotic disorders such as schizophrenia starting in childhood or adolescence is associated with worse outcomes.

Chapter 4
Case Finding and Screening

As discussed in Chapters 1 and 2, the early onset form of schizophrenia (EOS) is rare with a prevalence rate of approximately one in 10,000; however, schizophrenia occurs in approximately 1% of the adult population, and in about one third of cases, individuals begin experiencing psychotic symptoms in adolescence (Findling & Schulz, 2005; Kodish & McClellan, 2008). Schizophrenia is often preceded by subclinical symptoms and adjustment problems with a gradual deterioration in functioning over a period of months or years (Walker, Kestler, Hochman, & Bollini, 2005). More specifically, adults with a diagnosis of schizophrenia demonstrate increased social withdrawal, anxiety, academic difficulties, and thought problems that frequently begin in adolescence (Findling & Schulz, 2005). This suggests that school psychologists and other school-based mental health professionals are on the front line to identify and intervene for students who currently have or who are at risk of developing schizophrenia in the early stages of functional decline.

Before introducing strategies to identify early warning signs, this chapter discusses the early, prodromal (clinical high risk) stage of schizophrenia so that school mental health professionals can be attentive to these behavioral indicators among students. It also reviews assessment tools to screen and identify students at risk for developing either adult- or early-onset of schizophrenia (EOS) in order that supports and interventions can be introduced, thus altering the trajectory of the illness.

Prodromal Stage of Schizophrenia

The prodromal stage of schizophrenia "begins with the first changes in behavior and lasts up until the onset of psychosis" (Cornblatt, Lencz, & Kane, 2001, p. 32). It is marked by early symptoms that "precede the manifestation of the fully developed disorder or to a period of disturbance that represents a deviation from the person's previous experience and behavior" (Amminger, Leicester, Francey, & McGorry, 2005, p. 200). Prodromal symptoms are the first nonspecific indicators of active psychosis. In one study, the most frequently reported initial signs included restlessness,

H. Li et al., *Identifying, Assessing, and Treating Early Onset Schizophrenia at School*, Developmental Psychopathology at School, DOI 10.1007/978-1-4419-6272-0_4,

depression, anxiety, worrying, and difficulty with thinking or concentrating (Hafner & Maurer, 2006). In an Australian study, the most frequently reported symptoms included sleep disturbance, anxiety, social withdrawal, and irritability with an overall deterioration in role functioning (Yung & McGorry, 1996).

Establishing the onset of the prodrome is particularly challenging in EOS as the disorder tends to be more severe and the premorbid developmental anomalies more pronounced (Walker et al., 2005). In adult studies, the prodromal phase is organized into two stages: prepsychotic prodromal and psychotic prephase stage (Hafner & Maurer, 2006). The prepsychotic prodromal stage is the period from the first sign of illness until the first psychotic symptom and, on average, occurs over a 5-year period. The psychotic prephase is the period between the first positive symptom and the first psychiatric admission, and lasts on average about 1 year (Hafner & Maurer).

Of concern, however, is the fact that the constellation of symptoms that comprise the prodromal phase are not specific to schizophrenia. For example, the earliest signs of schizophrenia are similar to those of depressive episodes (Hafner & Maurer, 2006). With children, it is particularly important to consider a developmental perspective. For example, having an imaginary friend would be atypical for an adolescent, but 31% of 6- and 7-year-olds report having an imaginary friend (Taylor, Carlson, Maring, Gerow, & Charley, 2004). Also of paramount concern is the accurate identification of prodromal symptoms of schizophrenia to reduce misidentifying individuals as "false positives." Prodromal symptoms are relatively common in the general population, particularly young people, as a community-based survey indicated that nearly half of the sample (49%) endorsed two or more prodromal features (McGorry et al., 1995).

To date, most studies on the prodromal stage of schizophrenia have been conducted outside of the U.S. and have methodological shortcomings as they are based exclusively on retrospective reports from patients with schizophrenia and their families, thus making predictive accuracy uncertain as the reports are subject to distortion (Lee, McGlashan, & Woods, 2005). Few studies have validated and refined definitions of psychosis prodromal phase by prospective study, particularly with youth. In the last decade, there has been an exceptional increase in prodromal phase research; for example, 176 of 193 peer-reviewed articles on the prodromal stage have been published since 1995 (Addington et al., 2007). This exponential increase in information is attributed, in part, to research funding in 1999 by the National Institutes of Health, which focused on identification and early intervention in the prodromal phase of schizophrenia. This funding mechanism ultimately resulted in a prestigious research collaborative – the North American Prodrome Longitudinal Study (NAPLS) – that focuses on characterizing the prodromal stage and improving the accuracy of prospective prediction of initial psychosis. However, the limited prospective prodromal studies with U.S. populations raise questions about the feasibility of different screening and case identification strategies within this health care, educational, or legal systems context.

Case Finding

Case finding refers to the strategy of surveying all students in the general population to identify atypical developmental patterns. The routine surveillance methods are designed to recognize the presence of risk factors and/or warning signs that implicate the need for further screening and evaluation, thus acting as a method of primary prevention. Prevention of schizophrenia has become a critical issue as it is believed that there is a correlation between the duration of untreated psychosis (DUP) and the individual's prognosis (Cornblatt et al., 2001). Efforts to prevent the onset of schizophrenia are designed to "improve understanding of the mechanisms of disease onset and progression and to facilitate application of interventions before the illness takes hold, thereby reducing or preventing the devastating effects of schizophrenia" (Cannon et al., 2008, p. 28). A key challenge to preventing schizophrenia, however, is consistently identifying signs and symptoms that are precursors to the full disorder.

Case finding and early identification of prodromal states allows for early intervention services, yet the term "early intervention" in relation to the development of psychosis, and ultimately schizophrenia, is ambiguous. Larsen et al. (2001) have indicated that there are two points of early intervention strategies: (a) in the prodromal phase and (b) after the onset of psychosis. *Early intervention in the prodromal phase* would include primary prevention as it would focus on the general population and ultimately lead to a decrease in the incidence of the disorder. As an example, the Portland (Maine) Identification and Early Referral (PIER) program has the public health mission of reducing the incidence of psychotic illnesses by targeting people ages 12–35 years. This program educates stakeholders and the community about the early warning signs of psychosis, the importance of getting help early, and the benefits of early treatment (Downing & Spring, 2007). Preliminary findings indicate approximately 30 per 100,000 fewer first hospitalizations for psychosis compared with previous years (The Brown University Child and Adolescent Behavior Letter, 2007). *Early intervention after the onset of psychosis* refers to treatment after psychosis is present, to reduce the DUP, and ultimately reduce toxicity to the brain. Technically, interventions at this point would be referred to as secondary prevention. *Tertiary prevention* focuses on efforts to prevent relapse and has the primary focus of research in treatment. A graphic representation of the course of illness, and timelines for early intervention and prevention based on the work of Larsen et al. (2001) is included in Figure 4.1.

Comprehensive treatment is the focus of Chapter 7 and is particularly relevant for those who reach the diagnostic threshold of EOS, yet intervention in the prodromal stage is worthy of brief discussion in the context of case screenings as symptoms present in the prodromal stage are highly distressing to both the children and their families (Lee et al., 2005). According to Yung et al. (2007), "left unrecognized, untreated, or poorly treated, psychotic illnesses... not only lead to considerable personal and family distress and increased severity of illness, but also contribute to

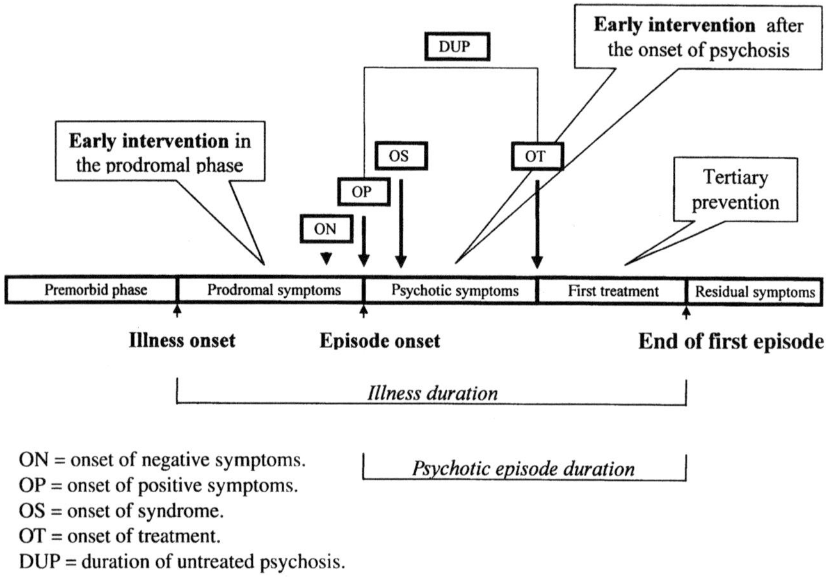

Fig. 4.1 The early course of schizophrenia figure (From Larsen et al., 2001, with permission)

poor academic performance, premature exit from school and higher education, unemployment, sustained disability, and premature death" (p. 633). Several studies suggest that early treatment, beginning after the onset of psychosis, results in reduced morbidity and a better quality of life outcome (Lee et al., 2005; Lieberman et al., 2001). In contrast, the longer the psychosis remains untreated, the poorer the prognosis. On average, a person may experience these symptoms between 1 and 2 years before treatment is implemented (Cornblatt, Lencz, & Obuchowski, 2002; Lieberman et al., 2001). The amount of time before treatment is implemented depends upon the accumulation of symptoms, help-seeking behavior, and the availability of mental health services (Hafner & Maurer, 2006). However, in a community-based sample of non-help-seeking adolescents, the mean age of onset of psychotic symptoms was 12.9 years and typically many years before individuals seek treatment, thus highlighting the need for early identification and treatment (Myles-Worsley et al., 2007). In a broad sense, secondary prevention is aimed at early detection and prompt treatment, as presently there is no cure for schizophrenia but rather efforts to reduce relapses, decrease family burden, and maintain the individual in the community (Ho et al., 2005).

Risk Factors

Although multiple risk factors for schizophrenia are documented (see Chapter 2 for a discussion of causes), no single factor has been identified as a powerful predictor:

rather, "there is the assumption that the disorder is caused by a complex interplay of biological, social, and psychological factors" (Yung et al., 2007, p. 636). Moreover, many of the childhood risk factors identified for adult-onset schizophrenia are also associated with affective psychosis and affective disorders (Hafner & Maurer, 2006). A number of studies have examined genetically high-risk individuals (e.g., children of parents with schizophrenia) with little recourse. For example, an estimated 10–15% percent of offspring of a parent with schizophrenia will become ill with a psychotic disorder, yet the great majority will not develop the disorder and the period of risk stretches over 2–3 decades (Walker et al., 2005). More recent approaches combine genetic risk factors with behavioral indicators to identify individuals that are at "ultra high risk" with more promising findings (discussed below). This risk paradigm allows the possibility that some individuals will not progress to full threshold psychotic disorder (Yung et al., 2005).

Population-based, prospective studies consistently indicate a developmental trajectory for children who later develop schizophrenia as adults, in that they demonstrate intellectual and language deficits, early motor delays, and subtle, nonspecific behavioral features (e.g., anxiety, hostility), (Welham, Isohanni, Jones, & McGrath, 2009). Other risk factors associated with prevalence and incidence rates include being male, having low cognitive ability, living in an urban area with low social capital, being an immigrant, or being from African–American or Asian–American heritage (see Chapter 3 for more information on these factors).

Warning Signs

Using risk factors alone is too narrow a basis for screening and preventive intervention for EOS, particularly since the behaviors listed as risk factors could be indicative of any number of psychopathologies. More recently, research has focused on early identification of individuals who are considered "ultra high risk" (UHR) for schizophrenia as they demonstrate genetic risk factors and early behavioral indicators, or warning signs (Yung et al., 2006; Yung et al., 2007). The ultra high risk (UHR) criteria are organized around three groups:

1. *Trait and state risk factor group*: Individuals in this group have a first-degree relative with a psychotic disorder or they have a schizotypal personality disorder and have experienced a significant decrease in functioning over the last year.
2. *Attenuated psychosis group*: Individuals in this group have experienced positive symptoms during the past year, but not with the intensity and frequency (subthreshold) required to be identified as psychosis.
3. *Brief limited intermittent psychotic syndrome* (BLIPS) *group*: Individuals in this group have experienced psychotic symptoms that have not lasted longer than a week and have spontaneously abated (Yung et al., 2006; Yung et al., 2007).

A list of early behavioral indicators and warning signs, based on the work of NAPLS, are included in Table4.1. Most prominently, longitudinal studies have

Table 4.1 Early Warning Signs of Risk for Psychosis (Modified from PRIME: (Yale PRIME Research Clinic, n.d.) http://www.med.yale.edu/psych/clinics/prime/prelig.html)

- Increased difficulty or worrisome decline in school, work, or social functioning
- New difficulty concentrating or thinking clearly
- Suspiciousness, mistrust, or uneasiness with others
- Unusual ideas, odd thinking, or behavior
- Changes in the way things look or sound
- Social withdrawal/isolation
- Emotional outbursts or lack of emotions
- Feeling depressed or anxious
- Withdrawal from friends and family
- Increased sensitivity to sensory experiences, or hearing unusual sounds or seeing things differently than usual
- Decline in self-care or personal hygiene
- Confusion about one's identity and future
- Feeling like their mind is playing tricks on them or that they are not in control of their ideas or thoughts

revealed that the greatest risk factor is self-reported delusional beliefs and hallucinatory experiences at the age of 11 (Poulton et al., 2000). In the study by Poulton and colleagues, children were asked the following questions about their beliefs and experiences: (a) Do you believe in mind reading or being psychic? Have other people ever read your mind? (b) Have you ever had messages sent to you through the television or radio? (c) Have you ever thought that people are following you or spying on you? (d) Have you heard voices other people can't hear? (e) Has something ever gotten inside your body or has your body changed in some way? (p. 1054). The children who responded positively to two of the five following questions were 16 times more likely to develop a schizophrenia-like psychosis by age 26 years.

Early indicators, as described here, can help school psychologists and other school-based mental health professionals know when to refer a student for additional psychiatric and community-based mental health services. However, once a student has been diagnosed with EOS, it is important for school personnel to monitor their illness and intervene when there are changes in their mental state with the psychosis becoming more prominent. From the work of Birchwood, Spenser, and McGovern (2000), information on warning signs of a psychotic *relapse* is also included in Table 4.2.

Screening and Assessment Tools

The recent interest in prevention and early intervention with schizophrenia has resulted in new assessment instruments, which are based on retrospective studies and are used to identify persons at a high enough risk for psychosis to differentiate diagnoses

Table 4.2 Early Signs of Psychotic Relapse (Reprinted with permission from Birchwood et al. (2000))

Thinking/perception	Feelings	Behaviors
Thoughts are racing	Feeling helpless or useless	Difficulty sleeping
Senses seem sharper	Feeling afraid of going crazy	Speech comes out jumbled filled with odd words
Thinking you have special powers	Feeling sad or low	Talking or smiling to yourself
Thinking that you can read other peoples minds	Feeling anxious and restless	Acting suspiciously as if being watched
Receiving personal messages from the TV or radio	Feeling increasingly religious	Behaving oddly for no reason
Having difficulty making decisions	Feeling like you're being watched	Spending time alone
Experiencing strange sensations	Feeling isolated	Neglecting your appearance
Preoccupied about one or two things	Feeling tired or lacking energy	Acting like you are somebody else
Thinking you might be somebody else	Feeling confused or puzzled	Not seeing people
Seeing visions or things other cannot see	Feeling forgetful or far away	Not eating
Thinking people are talking about you	Feeling in another world	Not leaving the house
Thinking people are against you	Feeling strong and powerful	Behaving like a child
Having more nightmares	Feeling unable to cope with everyday tasks	Refusing to do simple requests
Having difficulty concentrating	Feeling like you are being punished	Drinking more
Thinking bizarre things	Feeling like you cannot trust other people	Smoking more
Thinking your thoughts are controlled	Feeling irritable	Movements are slow
Hearing voices	Feeling like you do not need sleep	Unable to sit down for long
Thinking that a part of you has changed shape	Feeling guilty	Behaving aggressively

and justify early intervention (Hafner & Maurer, 2006). These instruments focus on the areas of attenuated positive symptoms (APS), which are typically demonstrated in the later part of the prodromal phase, and basic symptoms (BS), which are the trouble disturbances within the self that are associated with subjective complaints of emotional distress, difficulty concentrating, and avolition/apathy. A comprehensive review of prospective assessment tools for the prodromal phase was organized by Olsen and Rosenbaum (2006) and includes scales that focus on both APS and BS. The psychometric properties of two semi-structured interview instruments focusing on the APS, three that focus on BS, and four screening instruments are reviewed below.

Assessment Tools for the Attenuated Positive Symptoms of the Prodromal Stage

The two following assessment tools, the *Comprehensive Assessment of At Risk Mental States* (CAARMS) and the *Structured Interview of Prodromal Syndromes* (SIPS), assess APS and have been the most thoroughly studied instruments to date. Predictive validity studies of these two tools indicate that approximately 40–54% of those identified transition to full psychosis within a year (Loewy, Bearden, Johnson, Raine, & Cannon, 2005). In a comparison of these instruments, the *SIPS* relies more on recent symptoms and acute aggravation, and the psychosis threshold is lower. In the *CAARMS*, there is more emphasis on stable and persistent symptoms (Olsen & Rosenbaum, 2006). The instruments have primarily been used for research purposes and can serve as a template for understanding early signs. They are described more thoroughly below.

Comprehensive Assessment of At Risk Mental States (CAARMS; Yung et al., 2005). The *CAARMS* is a semi-structured interview developed at the Personal Assistance and Crisis Evaluation (PACE) clinic in Australia. This scale assesses psychopathology that may indicate the imminent development of psychotic disorders and determines if an individual is at "ultra high risk" (UHR) for psychotic disorders (Yung et al., 2006).

The scale is organized into seven symptom subscales, and on several of the subscales, both subjective and objective observation are rated. The subscales cover the following aspects: Positive symptoms, Cognitive change, Emotional disturbance, Negative symptoms, Behavioral change, Motor physical change, and General psychopathology. The dimensions measured are as follows: disorders of thought content, perceptual abnormalities, conceptual disorganization, motor disturbances, disorders of emotion and affect, impaired energy, and impaired tolerance to normal stress. This instrument has been translated into four languages, and the *Youth Psychosis At Risk Questionnaire* (Y-PARQ; Ord, Myles-Worsely, Blailes, & Ngirlmau, 2004) has been constructed as a screening questionnaire based on the *CAARMS*.

The *CAARMS* has demonstrated good discriminant validity and excellent interrater reliability (ICC in the range of 0.62–0.93 with only one subscale below 0.7). Sensitivity, or the ability to predict psychosis in all tested individuals, was 83% at 6 months, and specificity, or the percentage of all tested individuals who do not have this illness, was 74% at 6 months. The *CAARMS* has been able to differentiate between a control group and a UHR group, and high *CAARMS* scores in a UHR group have been significantly associated with onset of psychotic disorder (Yung et al., 2005).

Structured Interview of Prodromal Syndromes (SIPS; Miller et al., 2003). The *SIPS* is a semi-structured diagnostic interview designed for trained clinicians to distinguish prodromal syndromes from psychosis. The *SIPS* includes five components: a 19-item Scale of Prodromal Syndromes (SOPS), a checklist for the Criteria of Prodromal Symptoms (COPS), Global Assessment of Functioning, DSM-IV schizotypal personality disorder checklist, and a family history of mental illness (see Table4.3). In addition, it has an operational definition of psychosis onset – Presence of Psychotic Syndrome (POPS). The *SIPS* has been translated into 15 different languages.

Table 4.3 Organization of the *SIPS* and the *SOPS* and Listing of Associating Acronyms (Miller et al., 2003)

Structured interview for prodromal syndromes (SIPS)
Measures
Scale of prodromal symptoms (SOPS)
Schizotypal personality disorder checklist (DSM-IV)
Family history questionnaire
Global assessment of functioning scale (GAF)
Criteria
Presence of psychotic syndrome (POPS)
Criteria of prodromal syndromes (COPS)
Brief intermittent psychotic symptom syndrome (BIPS)
Attenuated positive symptom syndrome (APS)
Genetic risk and deterioration syndrome (GRD)
Scale of prodromal symptoms (SOPS)
Positive symptoms
Unusual thought content/delusional ideas
Suspiciousness/persecutory ideas
Grandiosity
Perceptual abnormalities / hallucinations
Disorganized communication
Negative symptoms
Social anhedonia
Avolition
Expression of emotion
Experience of emotions and self
Ideational richness
Occupational functioning
Disorganization symptoms
Odd behavior and appearance
Bizarre thinking
Trouble with focus and attention
Personal hygiene
General Symptoms
Sleep disturbance
Dysphoric mood
Motor disturbances
Impaired tolerance to normal stress

Among the five components, the SOPS measure the severity of prodromal symptoms and changes over time. It has four subscales – Positive, Negative, Disorganization, and General Symptoms scales. The Positive subscale is made up of five domains: unusual thought content/delusional ideas, suspiciousness/persecutory ideas, grandiosity, perceptual abnormalities/hallucination, and conceptual disorganization. Currently, the Positive subscale is used to make prodromal diagnosis and the other three subscales measure the severity of symptoms once the diagnosis is established. The COPS define three types of prodromal syndromes – Brief Intermittent Psychotic Symptom, Attenuated Positive Syndrome, and Genetic Risk and Deterioration. The symptom descriptions, onset, and duration of the three prodromal syndromes are presented in Table 4.4.

Reliability and validity data indicate excellent interrater reliability and predictive validity – resulting in it being the prodromal assessment tool of the NAPLS research collaborative. Specifically, the interrater agreement in making diagnostic judgments regarding the presence of the prodromal for schizophrenia reaches 93% (Miller et al., 2003). The SOPS rating scale has high reliability (ICC values at 0.95 for the total score and above 0.75 for all four subscales – Positive, Negative, Disorganized, and General Symptoms subscales). Sensitivity (percentage of all tested individuals who have developed this illness) was 100% at 6, 12, and 24 months; and specificity (percentage of all tested individuals who have not developed have this illness) was 71%, 74%, and 73% at 6, 12, and 24 months.

Assessment Tools for the Basic Symptoms of the Prodromal Stage

The instruments designed to assess basic symptoms (BS) focus more on the subtle, often only self-perceived, changes that occur during the prodromal decline. The deterioration is often associated with subjective complaints of emotional distress, difficulty concentrating or sleeping, irritability, and avolition/apathy. Psychotic symptoms typically gradually evolve and worsen, thus, the subjective nature of psychotic symptoms needs to be considered – particularly since there is a growing consensus that the "ultra high risk" and "basic symptoms" approaches are complementary to detecting different prodromal stages (Phillips et al., 2005). The following assessment tools focus on the subjective reports of cognitive, affective, and social disturbances that precede the first psychotic episode.

Bonn Scale for the Assessment of Basic Symptoms (BSABS; Gross, Huber, Klosterketter, Linz & Bonner, 1987). The *BSABS* was published in Germany in 1987 based on the work of Huber and colleagues (Klosterketter, Hellmich, Steinmeyer, & Schultze-Lutter, 2001). It is a 92-item semi-structured interview that explores subjective disturbances that are presumed to be the phenotype or manifestations of underlying deficits linked to schizophrenia. The items are organized into the following subscales: Dynamic Deficiency (changes in sleep, tolerance of stress, experience of emotions, phobias); Disturbances of Thought, Perception, and Motor Action (perseverative thoughts or memory disturbances, sensitivity to light or sound, and loss of automatic skills); Coenaesthesias (impaired bodily sensations); Disturbances of the Central Autonomic Nervous System; and Sleep Disturbances (Klosterkotter et al., 2001).

In a nearly 10-year longitudinal study, 70% of the identified patients went on to develop schizophrenia (sensitivity 0.98, specificity 0.59; Klosterkotter et al., 2001). This instrument demonstrates good reliability as measured by ICC (0.95–0.99) when compared to the Positive and Negative Syndrome Scale (PANSS), and 86%

Table 4.4 Structured Interview of Prodromal Syndromes (SIPS): Criteria of Prodromal Syndromes: Symptoms, Onset, and Duration (From Miller et al. (2003))

Prodromal criteria	Symptoms/descriptions	Ratings	Onset	Duration
Brief intermittent psychotic symptom syndrome	Frank psychotic symptoms that do not meet presence of psychotic syndromes criteria	A score of 6 on one or more of the 5 SOPS positive items in the psychotic range	Within past 3 months	Several minutes per day and once per month
Attenuated positive symptom syndrome	Mild psychotic symptoms that are not at a psychotic level of intensity (unusual thought content (paranoid, grandiose, perceptual abnormalities and disorganized speech with a score of 3, 4, or 5, but not reaching 6 – psychotic level) Perceptual abnormalities include hearing odd noises (more mild ones: banging, clicking, ringing, dogs barking when there are dogs present, name being called when no one has called) More severe ones: hearing sounds/voices that seem far away of rumbled, seeing colors differently, flashes of light or geographic shapes, seeing shadows out of corner of eyes or ghostlike figures Thought disorders include circumstantial or tangential speech, odd words or phrases, difficulty getting ideas crossed	A score of 3, 4, or 5 on one or more of the 5 SOPS positive times	Past year, symptoms increasing one or more points within the past year	Once per week for last month
Genetic risk and deterioration syndrome	First degree relative with any psychotic disorder, personally meeting the DSM-IV criteria for schizotypal personality	30% or more drop in functioning	Past year	Over the last month versus 1 year ago

of the items demonstrated an interrater reliability kappa >0.60 (Vollmer-Larsen, Handest, & Parnas, 2007). Prodromal symptoms as defined by *BSABS* have been incorporated into the *CAARMS* and *SIPS* early detection instruments (Klosterkotter et al., 2001).

Schizophrenia Proneness Instrument – Adult version (SPI-A; Schultze-Lutter, Ruhrmann, Picker, & Klosterkötter, 2006). The 34-item *SPI–A* is a semi-structured interview derived from the *BSABS* by cluster and confirmatory factor analyses. According to Schultze-Lutter et al. (2007), the *SPI–A* comprises six sub-scales that focus on the areas listed below, and demonstrated by the following behaviors:

1. Disturbances in affective functioning: Tolerance to certain stressors is impaired, less emotionally responsive and changes in general mood
2. Impairments in attention: Difficulty dividing attention between tasks, slowed processing, and difficulty with concentration and short-term memory
3. Basic cognitive disturbances: Indecisiveness with minor decision, thought blocking, disturbances in speech and immediate recall
4. Disturbances in self perception and experiences: Pressured thoughts, emotional confusion and increased reactivity, disturbance in sense of self and visual perception of others
5. Impaired bodily sensations: Perceptions disturbed in sensory processing
6. Sensitivity to perception: Hypersensitivity to light or sounds, bodily depersonalization (pp. s33–s34)

Preliminary results indicate good inter-rater reliability and good construct validity. Furthermore, 17% of those experiencing at least one basic symptom experienced psychosis within a 1-year period, suggesting good predictive validity (Olsen & Rosenbaum, 2006). Based on this scale, however, there are continued concerns for the need to develop criteria that distinguish between potential prodromal states and depression, though this study highlighted the importance of self-experienced cognitive deficits in the early detection of psychosis (Schultze-Lutter et al., 2006).

Early Detection Inventory (ERIraos; Hafner & Maurer; discussed in Wolwer et al., 2003). The *ERIraos* was developed as part of the German Research Network on Schizophrenia (GRNS), which coordinates research and care between more than 30 psychiatric departments and hospitals with more than 600 cooperating professionals. It was designed for the detection of disturbed mental states involving an increased risk of worsening or the development of psychotic illness based on retrospective studies. It is a two-step inventory to implement preventative strategies and optimize treatment for individuals with schizophrenia. The first part of the inventory is a 17-item checklist that functions as a screening instrument. If the screening score exceeds a cut-off level (i.e., score of 7 or above), then the second part of the instrument – a 110-item interview – is conducted, and this primarily focuses on detection, recognition, and early intervention in the prodromal stage (Wolwer et al., 2003). The *ERIraos* symptom list is divided into 12 sections that address changes in mood, personality, interest and drive, disturbance of sleep and appetite, dysfunctional behavior, anxiety and obsessive–compulsive symptoms, thought disorder, disorders of self and delusions, impaired bodily sensations (coenaesthesia), abnormal perceptions, and motor disorder. This tool is currently not published and validation of the screening instrument for early symptoms of psychosis is underway in Germany, Israel, and Italy (Hafner et al., 2005).

Screening Instruments

Identifying students who may be at risk for serious psychopathology can be achieved through population-based screening strategies; though to date few studies have conducted this type of research. Moreover, there is a significant challenge in identifying tools appropriate to screen for the decline in functioning associated with schizophrenia. An example of a preexisting, school-based screening strategy is the use of scholastic tests, such as the *Iowa Basic Skills Test*. Ho et al. (2005) concluded that such tests are *not* efficient screening methods for early detection of schizophrenia. However, declining performance on achievement tests could be used as a step to identify students in need of more intensive screening of behavioral indicators, such as social withdrawal, anxiety, and psychosis. This is particularly true if the decline occurs between the eighth and 11th grade – or ages 13 and 16, the onset of puberty, as it may be a precursor to the cognitive impairment that accompanies the first psychotic episode (Fuller et al., 2002). Similarly, declines in neurocognitive functioning may also indicate an important pattern of deterioration, particularly in the areas of verbal memory and general intellectual functioning – though additional research is needed to assess the predictive validity of these findings (Eastvold, Heaton, & Cadenhead, 2007). Thus, information readily available to school personnel (e.g., historical data from standardized achievement tests, cognitive assessments) may be of assistance when screening students for the development of serious psychopathology such as schizophrenia.

There are four prominent screening instruments designed as a time-efficient strategy to identify individuals with an increased risk of developing schizophrenia that need more intensive evaluation. The instruments reviewed below share adequate test-retest reliability, high convergent validity, and high inter-correlations, though they do not adequately distinguish between measures of depression, anxiety, and attention deficit disorders (Chang, Golembo, Maeda, Tsuji & Schiffman, 2008; Hafner & Maurer, 2006; Olsen & Rosenbaum, 2006). The screening tools include the *Youth Psychosis At Risk Questionnaire* (Y-PARQ), the *PRODscreen*, *SIPS screen*, and *Prodromal Questionnaire* (PQ). To date, however, all of the screening instruments are still being validated and are not systematically used in the general population – though there is the potential for their use in community-based settings (Myles-Worsley et al., 2007; Olsen & Rosenbaum, 2006).

Youth Psychosis At Risk Questionnaire (Y-PARQ; Ord et al., 2004). The *Y-PARQ*, based on the *CAARMS* (Yung et al., 2006), consists of 92 self-report (yes/no) items covering positive, affective, and negative symptoms. In a community-wide screening in Palau, high scores on the 24 most discriminating positive symptom items discriminated between normal and potentially prodromal adolescents. The *Y-PARQ* positive symptom score had a positive predictive value of 82% for identifying early psychosis, before reaching the UHR status (Ord et al., 2004). The researchers stated that a self-report questionnaire administered in high schools is an effective way to conduct community-wide screening of adolescents for prodromal symptomatology (Myles-Worsley et al., 2007).

PRODscreen (Heinimaa et al., 2003). The *PRODscreen*, developed in Finland, was designed to detect prodromal stages in adolescent and adult populations with elevated risk of psychosis. There are no reports on its use with children. It consists of 29 questions that can be administered through self-rating or self-report interview. The items focus on general functioning (e.g., current situation, changes during past year), general symptoms, and specific psychosis-like symptoms. It demonstrated concordant validity in that it correctly classified 77% of cases when compared to the SIPS. When used with a clinical sample, it is a reasonable predictor of prodrome – sensitivity of 80%, and specificity of 75% in the general population.

SIPS screen (Miller, Cicchetti, Markovich, McGlashan, & Woods, 2004). The *SIPS screen* is a brief self-report measure developed for screening persons at an increased risk for psychosis, based on the *Structured Interview of Prodromal Syndromes* (SIPS) discussed above. It contains 12 items that yielded a sensitivity of 0.90 and a perfect specificity in a sample of 36 patients compared with the SIPS evaluation. The authors indicated that it demonstrates promising psychometric properties, which present a novel and effective approach to early identification. It has not, however, been tested with nonclinical populations and has only been used to determine if the individual needs a more intensive assessment.

Prodromal Questionnaire (PQ; Loewy & Cannon, 2008). The *PQ* is a 92-item self-report, dichotomous (true/false) questionnaire organized into four major subscales: Positive, Negative, Disorganized, and General symptoms. The *PQ* is well-suited to preselect adolescent and adult individuals for more intensive interviewing and shows good preliminary validity in detecting individuals with prodromal or psychotic syndromes, as it has demonstrated 90% sensitivity and 49% specificity. There are no reports on its use with children. It is less sensitive, however, in determining the threshold between prodromal and full-blown psychosis. As it stands, the *PQ* can be used only for screening a clinical high risk population at specific prodrome clinics. The authors of the PQ have created a shorter, screening version (21 items); *The Prodromal Questionnaire-Brief Version (PQ-B)* with which to better assess levels of distress with the possibility of wider screening in nonclinical settings, such as schools and general medical facilities (Loewy & Cannon, 2010). The *PQ-B* is included in Table 4.5.

Summary and Conclusions

Research in the last decade has focused on identifying risk factors and warning signs for prodromal stages of schizophrenia. The prodrome begins with a pattern of behavioral symptoms and functional deterioration, yet it is both possible and plausible that covert internal experiences and cognitive and/or perceptual changes precede more

Table 4.5 *Prodromal Questionnaire – Brief version* (*PQ-B* ; Loewy & Cannon, 2008. Reprint with author permission). Please indicate whether you have had the following thoughts, feelings and experiences in the past month by checking "yes" or "no" for each item. Do not include experiences that occur only while under the influence of alcohol, drugs or medications that were not prescribed to you. If you answer "YES" to an item, also indicate how distressing that experience has been for you.

1. Do familiar surroundings sometimes seem strange, confusing, threatening or unreal to you?

   YES NO *If YES:* When this happens, I feel frightened, concerned, or it causes problems for me:

   Strongly disagree disagree neutral agree strongly agree

2. Have you heard unusual sounds like banging, clicking, hissing, clapping or ringing in your ears?

   YES NO *If YES:* When this happens, I feel frightened, concerned, or it causes problems for me:

   Strongly disagree disagree neutral agree strongly agree

3. Do things that you see appear different from the way they usually do (brighter or duller, larger or smaller, or changed in some other way)?

   YES NO *If YES:* When this happens, I feel frightened, concerned, or it causes problems for me:

   Strongly disagree disagree neutral agree strongly agree

4. Have you had experiences with telepathy, psychic forces, or fortune telling?

   YES NO *If YES:* When this happens, I feel frightened, concerned, or it causes problems for me:

   Strongly disagree disagree neutral agree strongly agree

5. Have you felt that you are not in control of your own ideas or thoughts?

   YES NO *If YES:* When this happens, I feel frightened, concerned, or it causes problems for me:

   Strongly disagree disagree neutral agree strongly agree

6. Do you have difficulty getting your point across, because you ramble or go off the track a lot when you talk?

   YES NO *If YES:* When this happens, I feel frightened, concerned, or it causes problems for me:

   Strongly disagree disagree neutral agree strongly agree

7. Do you have strong feelings or beliefs about being unusually gifted or talented in some way?

   YES NO *If YES:* When this happens, I feel frightened, concerned, or it causes problems for me:

   Strongly disagree disagree neutral agree strongly agree

8. Do you feel that other people are watching you or talking about you?

   YES NO *If YES:* When this happens, I feel frightened, concerned, or it causes problems for me:

   Strongly disagree disagree neutral agree strongly agree

9. Do you sometimes get strange feelings on or just beneath your skin, like bugs crawling?

   YES NO *If YES:* When this happens, I feel frightened, concerned, or it causes problems for me:

   Strongly disagree disagree neutral agree trongly agree

(continued)

Table 4.5 (continued)

10. Do you sometimes feel suddenly distracted by distant sounds that you are not normally aware of?

YES NO *If YES:* When this happens, I feel frightened, concerned, or it causes problems for me:

Strongly disagree disagree neutral agree strongly agree

11. Have you had the sense that some person or force is around you, although you couldn't see anyone?

YES NO *If YES:* When this happens, I feel frightened, concerned, or it causes problems for me:

Strongly disagree disagree neutral agree strongly agree

12. Do you worry at times that something may be wrong with your mind?

YES NO *If YES:* When this happens, I feel frightened, concerned, or it causes problems for me:

Strongly disagree disagree neutral agree strongly agree

13. Have you ever felt that you don't exist, the world does not exist, or that you are dead?

YES NO *If YES:* When this happens, I feel frightened, concerned, or it causes problems for me:

Strongly disagree disagree neutral agree strongly agree

14. Have you been confused at times whether something you experienced was real or imaginary?

YES NO *If YES:* When this happens, I feel frightened, concerned, or it causes problems for me:

Strongly disagree disagree neutral agree strongly agree

15. Do you hold beliefs that other people would find unusual or bizarre?

YES NO *If YES:* When this happens, I feel frightened, concerned, or it causes problems for me:

Strongly disagree disagree neutral agree strongly agree

16. Do you feel that parts of your body have changed in some way, or that parts of your body are working differently?

YES NO *If YES:* When this happens, I feel frightened, concerned, or it causes problems for me:

Strongly disagree disagree neutral agree strongly agree

17. Are your thoughts sometimes so strong that you can almost hear them?

YES NO *If YES:* When this happens, I feel frightened, concerned, or it causes problems for me:

Strongly disagree disagree neutral agree strongly agree

18. Do you find yourself feeling mistrustful or suspicious of other people?

YES NO *If YES:* When this happens, I feel frightened, concerned, or it causes problems for me:

Strongly disagree disagree neutral agree strongly agree

19. Have you seen unusual things like flashes, flames, blinding light, or geometric figures?

YES NO *If YES:* When this happens, I feel frightened, concerned, or it causes problems for me:

Strongly disagree disagree neutral agree strongly agree

(continued)

Table 4.5 (continued)

20. Have you seen things that other people can't see or don't seem to see?				
YES	NO	*If YES:* When this happens, I feel frightened, concerned, or it causes problems for me:		
Strongly disagree	disagree	neutral	agree	strongly agree
21. Do people sometimes find it hard to understand what you are saying?				
YES	NO	*If YES:* When this happens, I feel frightened, concerned, or it causes problems for me:		
Strongly disagree	disagree	neutral	agree	strongly agree

A cutoff score of 8 or more items deserve further evaluation.

overt behavioral indicators (Poulton et al., 2000). The prodromal phase is a unique window of opportunity where primary and secondary prevention meet, and by being aware of early warning signs and risk factors, school psychologists can play a unique role in improving the trajectory for those with schizophrenia. The information on risk factors and early warning signs in this chapter can serve as a foundation for screening students for more intensive evaluation and treatment, as ongoing functional decline in the school setting – academically and socially – can be an indicator that the student requires further assessment and connection to appropriate mental health services. "Ultimately a systematic approach toward diagnostic assessment and treatment monitoring will lead to a more timely initiation of appropriate treatment, better identification of risk factors, and safety concerns and improved outcomes" (Frazier et al., 2007, p. 986).

Assessment and screening tools that identify prodromal states can be critical in early intervention and prevention of psychotic episodes. Self-report questionnaire screening tools are an effective way to conduct community-wide screening of adolescents for prodromal or at-risk mental states, particularly with non-helping-seeking adolescents, as it is "an important adjunct to genetic high risk strategies for identifying early psychosis" (Myles-Worsley et al., 2007, p. 4; Ord et al., 2004). A major concern, however, is the nonspecific nature of the symptoms associated with schizophrenia, which are indistinguishable from other dimensions of psychopathology (Hafner et al., 2005). The risk status of stigmatizing individuals as "false positives" suggests the need for strict ethical practices. These ethical concerns must be balanced with the consequences of psychosis and its toxicity to the brain.

Chapter 5
Diagnostic Assessment

As indicated in Chapter 1, early onset schizophrenia (EOS) cases appear before age 18 (Remschmidt, 2002), meeting the diagnostic criteria established for adults. The diagnostic assessment of EOS can be challenging for mental health professionals. First, many symptoms of EOS may also appear in other psychiatric disorders such as ADHD, autism, depression, or anxiety. Second, some warning signs or at-risk behaviors of EOS can last several months or a few years as nonspecific psychological, behavioral, emotional, and social disturbances of varying intensity, and sometimes they can be difficult to distinguish from characteristics related to normal child or adolescent development (Woods, Miller, McGlashan, 2001). Third, parents, teachers, social workers, psychologists, or primary care doctors may not be familiar with symptoms or warning signs of EOS. And fourth, stigma associated with this debilitating illness creates reluctance and delay in active help seeking. A diagnosis of schizophrenia is usually made by a child psychiatrist based on the *DSM-IV-TR* criteria (APA, 2000). However, school psychologists are on the frontline in detecting at-risk behaviors for severe mental illnesses like EOS. Knowledge of the EOS diagnostic criteria, symptom onset, developmental course, and assessment instruments is essential in establishing an accurate diagnosis.

Diagnostic Criteria

The diagnosis of schizophrenia is based on the criteria of *DSM-IV-TR*. The full diagnostic criteria are presented in Table 5.1. In brief, the diagnostic symptoms for schizophrenia include hallucinations (a phenomena of a person reporting sensory perceptions which are not observed and confirmed by other people in the same setting, hallucinations can be auditory, visual, olfactory, tactile, or mixed type), delusions (a belief that is false), disorganized speech (incoherent and circumstantial), grossly disorganized behavior, and negative symptoms. The negative symptoms include withdrawal, flat affect, avolition (a lack of effort to act on one's own behalf or to engage in behaviors directed at accomplishing a purpose), or alogia (a disruption in thought process reflected in the person's speech, such as a poverty of speech or poverty of content).

H. Li et al., *Identifying, Assessing, and Treating Early Onset Schizophrenia at School*, Developmental Psychopathology at School, DOI 10.1007/978-1-4419-6272-0_5,

Table 5.1 DSM IV-TR Diagnostic Criteria for Schizophrenia (Reprinted with permission from the Diagnostic and Statistical Manual of Mental Disorders, Fourth Edition, Text Revision, (Copyright 2000, American Psychiatric Association)

A. Characteristic symptoms: Two (or more) of the following, each present for a significant portion of time during a 1-month period (or less if successfully treated):
   (1) Delusions
   (2) Hallucinations
   (3) Disorganized speech (e.g., frequent derailment or incoherence)
   (4) Grossly disorganized or catanotic behavior
   (5) Negative symptoms, i.e., affective flattening, alogia, or avolition
   Note: Only one criterion A symptom is required if delusions are bizarre or hallucinations consist of a voice keeping up a running commentary on the person's behavior or thoughts, or two or more voices conversing with each other.

B. Social/occupational dysfunction: For a significant portion of the time since the onset of the disturbance, one or more major areas of functioning such as work, interpersonal relations, or self-care are markedly below the level achieved prior to the onset (or when the onset is in childhood or adolescence, failure to achieve expected level of interpersonal, academic, or occupational achievement)

C. Duration: Continuous signs of the disturbance persist for at least 6 months. This 6-month period must include at least 1 month of symptoms (or less if successfully treated that meet criterion A (i.e., active-phase symptoms) and may include periods of prodromal or residual symptoms. During these prodromal or residual periods, the signs of the disturbance may be manifested by only negative symptoms or two or more symptoms listed in criterion A present in an attenuated form (e.g., odd beliefs, unusual perceptual experiences)

D. Schizoaffective and mood disorder exclusion: Schizoaffective and mood disorder with psychotic features have been ruled out because either (1) no major depressive, manic, or mixed episodes have occurred concurrently with the active-phase symptoms; or (2) if mood episodes have occurred during active-phase symptoms, their total duration has been brief relative to the duration of the active and residual periods

E. Substance/general medical condition exclusion; the disturbance is not due to the direct physiological effects of a substance (e.g., a drug of abuse, a medication) or a general medical condition.

F. Relationship to a pervasive developmental disorder: if there is a history of autistic disorder or another pervasive developmental disorder, the additional diagnosis of schizophrenia is made only if prominent delusions or hallucinations are also present for at least a month (or less if successfully treated)

Classification of longitudinal course (can be applied only after at least 1 year has elapsed since the initial onset of active-phase symptoms):
   Episodic with interepisode residual symptoms (episodes are defined by the reemergence of prominent psychotic symptoms); also specify if: With prominent negative symptoms
   Episodic with no interepisode residual symptoms
   Continuous (prominent psychotic symptoms are present throughout the period of observation); also specify if: With prominent negative symptoms
   Single episode in partial remission; also specify if: With prominent negative symptoms
   Single episode in full remission
   Other or unspecified pattern

Functional decline and duration of symptoms also need to be considered when making a diagnosis.

According to *DSM-IV-TR,* there are five schizophrenia subtypes: Paranoid Type, Disorganized Type, Catatonic Type, Undifferentiated Type, and Residual Type.

Among the five subtypes, the Paranoid Subtype is regarded as the least severe and the Disorganized Subtype as the most severe (APA, 2000). The subtypes are also classified into three dimensional descriptors for current and lifetime symptomatology of schizophrenia – psychotic, disorganized, and negative dimensions. The psychotic dimension includes symptoms of delusions and hallucinations, which are also called positive symptoms. The disorganized dimension includes disorganized speech, disoriented behavior, and inappropriate affect. The negative dimension includes the aforementioned negative symptoms such as withdrawal, flat affect, avolition, or alogia. Based on the severity of a person's symptoms, an absent, mild, moderate, or severe specification is assigned to each of the three dimensions for either or both the current episode (past 6 months) or/and the lifetime course of the disorder (APA, 2000).

Symptom Onset

Late adolescence to mid-30s is a time when symptoms of schizophrenia are most likely to appear (see Chapter 3 for further discussion of the incidence, prevalence, and onset). Those who were diagnosed as having schizophrenia before age 18 are classified as early onset schizophrenia (EOS) and those who developed schizophrenia at or before age 12 have child onset schizophrenia (COS) or very early onset schizophrenia (VEOS). The clinical manifestations of symptoms are similar in children and adolescents. There are two types of symptoms characteristic of schizophrenia: positive symptoms and negative symptoms. Positive symptoms are manifested as behavioral overrepresentation – hallucination, fixed delusional beliefs, and disorganized thought process. Negative symptoms tend to be manifested as behavioral deficits, including blunt affect, lack of energy, poor social communication, and paucity of speech or thoughts (APA, 2000). In addition, negative symptoms usually appear earlier than positive symptoms. EOS is often associated with hallucination, thought disorder, and flat affect. When hallucination is reported among children and adolescents, visual hallucinations such as shadows and dots are more common than auditory hallucinations (APA). Eggers and Bunk (1997) indicate that it is difficult to diagnose delusion and hallucination symptoms before age nine as these symptoms are not as elaborate as those observed in older children. Systematic delusions (false beliefs that have certain themes) are also reportedly less common in COS as they require advanced cognitive and abstract ability. Thus, the delusional contents may change over time as children mature. Furthermore, youth with EOS are more likely to demonstrate significant deficits in communication, with loose association, illogical thinking, and poor communication skills (Caplan, 1994).

Developmental Course

EOS is best understood as a neurodevelopmental disorder (Lewis & Levitt, 2002). As presented in Table 5.2, the clinical course of EOS is characterized by three phases, based on the symptom presentation and treatment response – prodromal,

Table 5.2 Clinical Course of Schizophrenia (Adapted From Kodish & McClellan, 2008)

Phases	Symptoms	Duration
Prodrome	Mild positive symptoms (changes in the way things look or sound)	Weeks up to 3 years
	Vague and increased feelings of uneasiness, depression, anxiety	
	Stress vulnerability	
	Cognitive and academic difficulties	
	Social isolation/disruption and deterioration in role functioning	
	Emotional outbursts or lack of emotion	
	Increased idiosyncratic or bizarre preoccupations	
	Suspiciousness of/lack of trust of others	
	Difficulty concentrating or thinking clearly	
	Poor hygiene	
Acute	Sharp functional decline and increase of hallucinations, delusions, and disorganized speech/behavior	1–6 months
	These symptoms can appear suddenly.	
Residual	Lower intensity or frequency of positive symptoms (with medication)	A few months to life time
	Continued impairment due to negative symptoms (social withdrawal, depression, avolition, etc.)	
	Feeling or behaving listless, trouble concentrating	
	Symptoms similar to prodromal phase	
	Subsequent acute episodes (one or more episodes), increased residual symptoms after each relapse	
	With no symptoms before the first episode of schizophrenia, few or no symptoms may be experienced after the first acute phase	

acute, and residual phases. Developmentally many individuals who have developed EOS begin to manifest deficits in different domains at an early age. According to Walker, Kestler, Bollini, and Hochman (2004), motor abnormality has been observed in young children who later on developed schizophrenia. These motor problems include delays in motor development, bimanual manipulation (being able to use both hands), and walking. It should be noted that impaired motor development is also observed in children at risk for a variety of other disorders, such as learning disabilities. An array of poor social behaviors has also been reported among youth with EOS. For instance, a cohort study of participants born in 1946 including individuals who subsequently developed schizophrenia showed that at ages four and six, they were observed to be more likely to play alone; at 13 years, they were less confident; and at 155 years, they were rated by teachers as more anxious in social situations (Jones, Rodgers, Murray, & Marmot, 1994). Other large-scale international studies also showed that poor social relations were evident at ages 16–17 years in individuals who subsequently developed schizophrenia (Davidson et al., 1999; Malmberg, Lewis, David, & Allebeck, 1998). In addition, they had fewer friends, preferred to socialize in small groups, were more sensitive, and were less likely to have romantic relationships. However, such problems may not be prodromal features (early warning signs) of schizophrenia, as they could persist in some individuals up to a decade. Thus, it is not clear whether these social abnormalities reflect actual illness process or whether they represent psychological risk factors for schizophrenia (Lewis & Levitt, 2002).

As indicated earlier, youth with EOS tend to experience negative symptoms (such as affective flattening, alogia, or avolition) early in the illness, presented as prodromal features before suffering positive symptoms (such as hallucination and/or delusion). In addition, some children and youth at risk of developing EOS manifest cognitive and social function decline, loss of interest in school, deterioration in hygiene, unusual behavior, outbursts of anger, and social isolation and withdrawal (APA, 2000). Adolescents at this phase may turn to illicit drugs in an effort to manage the frightening symptoms. These cognitive, social, emotional, and behavioral problems may cause confusion among family members, teachers, school psychologists, and other mental health professionals as they may be precursors of schizophrenia, or other mental disorders, or even part of normal development. It is highly likely that a child experiencing the aforementioned symptoms be referred to a school psychologist for an evaluation of learning disabilities, emotional disturbance, ADHD, autism, conduct disorder, or mental retardation, before a formal referral is made for a comprehensive psychiatric evaluation.

Schizophrenia is an episodic illness with symptoms that vary in intensity overtime. The course of schizophrenia is different for each individual (Hollis, 1995). In general, individuals with an early age at onset tend to demonstrate greater social deficits, lower levels of employment, "poorer premorbid adjustment, lower educational achievement, more evidence of structural brain abnormalities, more prominent negative signs and symptoms, more evidence of cognitive impairment as assessed with neuropsychological testing, and a worse outcome" (APA, 2000, p. 308).

The overall prognosis of individuals with schizophrenia also varies. A constellation of factors are associated with its better outcome. These factors include good premorbid adjustment, acute onset, later age onset, good insight, being female, fewer stressful life events, timely and appropriate medication after first episode of illness, strong family support, and absence of family history of schizophrenia. Poor prognosis is predicted by low premorbid functioning, family history of nonaffective psychotic illnesses, poor therapeutic resources, lack of engagement in services, severe symptoms during acute phases, higher rates of negative symptoms, and an onset before adolescence (APA, 2000).

Associated Features

Children and adolescents with EOS may experience challenges before and after they were diagnosed as having EOS. At the prolonged prodromal or at risk stage before they receive a clinical diagnosis of EOS, children may manifest behaviors which may not be specific to schizophrenia. In addition to the behavioral problems presented in the Developmental Course section of this chapter, these children may also experience social phobia, obsession and compulsivity, and academic decline. Poor sleeping patterns or loss of interest in eating are also observed in some youth. Youth or their teachers may complain about their difficulty in concentration, attention, and memory. Motor abnormalities are among the earlier signs of neurodevelopmental problems in individuals with schizophrenia, and they are more pronounced in early onset cases (Burke, Androustsos, Jogia, Byrne, & Frangou, 2008). Further, some individuals with EOS have symptoms of grimacing, posturing, unusual mannerism, ritualistic, or stereotypical behavior (APA, 2000). Deficits in recognizing, assessing, experiencing emotions, and processing of emotional facial expressions are observed in individuals with EOS (Seiferth et al., 2009). Such deficits may affect effective social interaction and subjective well-being. School psychologists should be aware of the complicated features related to EOS that could complicate the diagnostic process when evaluating students for special education services.

Age Specific Features

EOS and COS share similar symptoms when compared with adult onset schizophrenia. Both EOS and COS have "insidious onset, more severe premorbid neurodevelopmental abnormalities, more frequent terrifying visual hallucination, constant inappropriate or blunted affects, higher rate of familial psychopathology, minor response to treatment, and poorer outcome" (Margari et al., 2008, p. 825). However, younger children with EOS may experience more visual than auditory hallucinations and such hallucinations are typically less elaborate than those of older adolescents and adults with schizophrenia (APA, 2000). Retrospective and clinical studies (e.g., Hollis, 1995) indicate that the frequency and severity of speech and language deficits increase as age of onset decreases. In other words, the earlier the onset of schizophrenia is, the more severe the speech and language deficits are.

Gender Related Features

According to *DSM-IV-TR* (APA, 2000) and several researchers (e.g., Lindamer, Lohr, Harris, & Jeste, 2004; Maurer & Hafner, 1995; Riecher et al., 1990), on average, females are diagnosed with schizophrenia 2–10 years later than males. While both male and females had a peak onset at age 15–25 years, more male incidences appear at that age period than females. Lindamer et al. (2004) reported that among those who developed schizophrenia below age 25 years, 61% were males. Therefore, it can be said that in younger age groups, the risk is higher for males than for females. No gender difference is conclusive in the life-time risk of developing schizophrenia.

Research findings of gender differences of psychotic symptoms are not consistent. Some researchers report that male patients tend to show psychotic symptoms at an earlier age than female patients (e.g., DeLisi, 1992). However, Eggers and Bunk (1997) found in their longitudinal follow-up study that all the female patients manifested psychotic symptoms by the age of 15 years, whereas 100% of boys showed psychotic symptoms by the age 18 years.

Speech disturbances have been identified as a characteristic trait of schizophrenia. For example, Walder et al. (2006) report significant gender differences in grammar, phonological processing, and semantics in that females with schizophrenia performed significantly better than their male counterparts. These results are consistent with findings that indicate males with schizophrenia demonstrate more impaired verbal learning and verbal fluency (e.g., Gourovitch, Goldberg, Weinberger, 1996).

Differential Diagnosis

As indicated earlier, some complicated clinical symptoms are not only associated with EOS, but also with other psychiatric illnesses. Thus, differential diagnosis must be taken into consideration before a diagnosis of EOS is made when evaluating children and adolescents who experience schizophrenia like symptoms. In addition, children with EOS frequently get many other diagnoses before they get a diagnosis of EOS. The following presents occasions when EOS should be ruled out as well as disorders and their differentiating features from EOS, based on *DSM-IV-TR* and recent research findings.

Psychotic Disorder due to a General Medical Condition. EOS should be ruled out if a comprehensive evaluation including history, physical examination, or lab tests reveal medical conditions like brain tumor or Cushing's syndrome (APA, 2000).

Substance-Induced (Psychotic Disorder, Delirium, or Persisting Dementia). EOS should be ruled out if drug abuse, a certain medication, or exposure to toxic materials are associated with the emergence of psychotic symptoms. However, as this population has a disproportionately high risk for substance abuse, it can be challenging to determine if the psychotic symptoms precede the substance abuse or originate from the abuse (APA, 2000).

Mood Disorder with Psychotic Features. EOS is ruled out if "psychotic symptoms occur exclusively during periods of mood disturbance" (APA, 2000, p. 310). However, this differential diagnosis can be challenging as mood disturbances are also often comorbid with EOS.

Schizoaffective Disorder. Schizoaffective Disorder is differentiated from Schizophrenia (not specific to EOS) in that a mood episode must be present for an extended amount of time during the total duration of positive symptoms of schizophrenia. In addition, positive symptoms such as delusion and/or hallucination must be present for at least 2 weeks in the absence of prominent mood symptoms (APA, 2000).

Schizophreniform Disorder. This disorder differentiates with Schizophrenia in the duration of illness. For Schizophrenia, the symptoms (including prodromal or residual symptoms) have to be present for at least 6 months. For Schizohphreniform Disorder, the symptoms should last at least a month but less than 6 months. In addition, no functioning decline is required in diagnosing Schizophreniform Disorder (APA, 2000).

Pervasive Developmental Disorders (PDD). PDD differs from EOS or COS in the age of onset. Many PDD cases such as autism usually are identified before age three while the youngest COS cases so far have been found among children in 5 or 6 years of age. Severe speech impairment and prominent stereotypical behaviors are present in children with PDD, however, hallucinations and delusions may not be present in most PDD, cases. If children with PDD manifest positive symptoms, a comorbid EOS can be added to the current diagnosis of PDD. The impaired generalized intellectual ability and negative symptoms of COS and EOS may make it difficult to differentiate them from children with PDD, who also experience impaired cognitive impairment and social communication skills (Kodish & McClellan, 2007).

Obsessive Compulsive Disorder. Children and youth with OCD differ from those with EOS in that the former group is able to realize and acknowledge their irrational beliefs and rituals resulted from extreme anxiety and worry about what would happen to themselves and/or their family members. The EOS group, however, is noted for their lack of insight and loss of touch with reality (Kodish & McClellan, 2008).

Other Diagnosis. Youth with conduct problems, emotional disturbance, or maltreatment history may occasionally report psychotic like symptoms. These symptoms, however, may be more dissociative and anxiety driven. Sometimes such symptoms are situation specific, coincided with attention seeking behaviors or angry outbursts. These youth who manifest atyptical psychotic-like behaviors may have lower rates of bizarre behaviors and thought disorder. Therefore, even with some degree of positive symptoms, they may thereby have conduct disorder or emotional disturbance, rather than EOS (Kodish & McClellan, 2008).

Developmental, Health, and Family History

An important step of understanding and diagnosing EOS starts with a thorough interview with the child and significant people in the child's life regarding his or her developmental and medical history. Mental health professionals should also inquire about the family psychiatric history, as indicated in Chapter 2; a positive family history of schizophrenia may increase a child's risk of developing EOS.

Prenatal, Perinatal, and Postnatal Risk Factors

A large body of data has provided evidence of enhanced risk of schizophrenia following prenatal, perinatal, and postnatal exposure to infection with lead or various viral pathogens, including influenza, rubella, measles, herpe simplex, toxoplasma gondii, as well as infection with bacterial pathogens and genital and/or reproductive infections (Brown et al., 2001; Brown et al., 2004; Opler, & Susser, 2005; Patterson, 2007). Therefore, a thorough examination of the mother's pregnancy and labor history should be conducted in the diagnostic process. Please refer to Chapter 2 for more information on prenatal, perinatal, and postnatal risk factors of schizophrenia.

Developmental Milestones

Children and youth who have developed EOS show different early developmental trajectories. Some individuals with EOS may show minor abnormalities (e.g., cognitive, language, social, or motor functioning) during childhood and these abnormalities deteriorat over the years, while others with EOS display severe behavioral abnormalities during childhood, and these abnormalities would remain relatively stable overtime (Corcoran et al., 2003; Vourdas, Pipe, Corrigall, & Frangou, 2003). Still others who have the illness might have had an essentially normal development through childhood. Developmental milestones are crucial information to gather at the initial stages of assessment to facilitate the diagnosis.

As indicated in Chapter 6, developmental delays in speech and language production has been reported in individuals with COS and EOS (Kolvin, Ounsted, Humphrey, & McNay, 1971). In fact, language impairment is found to be more common in EOS than in youth with other psychiatric illnesses (Hollis, 1995). The pattern of language impairment (language production and/comprehension) also varies with age of onset in that it is more common in COS than those with EOS. Youth with EOS are also found to have delayed speech milestone, as well as more reading and spelling difficulties compared with normal controls (Vourdas et al., 2003). Males with EOS reportedly experience more problems with regard to speech development than females. The communication of many children who later develop schizophrenia is often referred to as odd or inappropriate. In some cases, children progress from a long-standing communication disorder to the insidious onset of thought disorder and disorganized behavior which are hallmarks of EOS (Hollis, 1995).

Medical History

As the trusted mental health professionals of parents, school psychologists can facilitate the assessment and diagnosis by collecting a thorough medical history of the child or adolescent during the initial phases of evaluation. Information about a child's current vision and hearing status should be collected. History of brain infection /injury, brain tumor, Cushing's disease, hyperthyroidism, syphilis, Vitamin B12 deficiency, or seizures should also be collected, as they can produce psychotic like symptoms (Kelsey, Newport, & Nemeroff, 2006).

Diagnostic History

EOS is a very complicated disorder, and it is difficult to diagnose accurately at a single time point. Therefore, an individual with EOS may over time have his or her diagnosis changed to and from schizophrenia (Kelsey et al., 2006). Furthermore, it is well known that full blown psychotic symptoms in schizophrenia are preceded by a prodromal phase of anywhere from weeks to 2 or 3 years. As indicated earlier in this chapter, children and adolescents at the prodromal or at-risk phase may display relatively unspecific symptoms to schizophrenia – including depression, anxiety, social withdrawal, subtle neurocognitive deficits, functional decline, behavioral and academic difficulties, and subtle positive symptoms. Therefore, many of these children or adolescents may have been receiving special education services at school setting or receiving outpatient treatment of psychiatric illnesses other than EOS.

Furthermore, as discussed in Chapter 3, psychiatric comorbidities are also common among individuals with schizophrenia. For example, anxiety and depressive symptoms are very common throughout the course of illness, with an estimated prevalence of 15% for panic disorder, 29% for posttraumatic stress disorder, 23% for obsessive-compulsive disorder, 50% for depression, and perhaps 47% of patients also have a lifetime diagnosis of comorbid substance abuse (Buckley, Miller, Lehrer, & Castle, 2009). Therefore, a careful examination of the history and timing of previous diagnoses may provide school psychologists and other mental health professionals with information and insights into the nature of a child's illness, thereby facilitating a more accurate diagnosis.

Indirect Assessment

Best and ethical practices in the diagnostic assessment of psychological and psychiatric disorders stipulate that the assessment be conducted with multiple informants using multiple types of assessment instruments and procedures. The assessment procedures familiar to school psychologists in assessing early warning signs and symptoms of EOS tend to fall into two categories – indirect assessment method and direct observational method. The former category includes rating scales and clinical interviews and the latter one involves the observation of the target behavior (s) at the moment when the behavior is occurring. The following introduces the two types of indirect assessment of EOS related symptoms – rating scales and interviews.

Rating Scales: Child Behavior Checklist (CBCL; Achenbach & Rescorla, 2001). The *CBCL* is a standardized parent-completed checklist of competencies and behavior problems of children and adolescents, 6–18 years of age. Teacher Report Form (TRF) and Youth Self-Report (YRS) versions are also available. The *CBCL/6-18* has 118 items that describe specific behavioral and emotional problems, along with two open-ended items for reporting additional problems. Parents rate their child on how true each item is now or within the past 6 months. *CBCL* has high interrater reliability of 0.93–0.96, and the internal consistency of the subscales ranges from 0.78 to 0.97. Adequate criterion validity has been established. The *CBCL/6-18*, TRF, and YSR include the following scales: Aggressive Behavior, Anxious/Depressed, Attention Problems, Rule-Breaking Behavior, Social Problems, Somatic Complaints, Thought Problems, and Withdrawn/Depressed. Muratori, Salvadori, D'Arcangelo, Viglione, and Picchi (2005) examined the premorbid behaviors of adolescent patients with EOS, anorexia patients, and healthy controls using *CBCL*. They found that youth with EOS showed significantly higher scores on all scales even before they developed EOS, relative to the control group; and only on some scales (social, thought and attention problems, and school competencies) relative to the anorexia group.

Behavior Assessment System for Children-II (BASC-II; Kamphaus & Reynolds, 2004). The *BASC-II* is used to determine youth's behavioral and emotional strengths and weaknesses based on information gathered from teachers, parents, and youth. Teacher Rating Scales (TRS) measure a child's strengths and problem behaviors in school setting. Teachers respond to descriptors of behaviors on a four-point scale of frequency from "Never" to "Almost Always." The TRS yields 15 primary scores (adaptability, aggression, anxiety, attention problems, atypicality, conduct problems, depression, functional communication, hyperactivity, leadership, learning problems, social skills, somatization, study skills, and withdrawal), and seven content scores (such as Anger Control, Executive Functioning, or Negative Emotionality). For the individual scales, the TRS has median test-retest reliability of 0.86 and 0.81 at child and adolescent levels (Kamphaus & Reynolds). Interrater reliability at child and adolescent levels for individual scales were 0.56 and 0.53. Convergent and discriminant validities of the scales were established in comparison with the *CBCL*-TRF and *Conners Teacher Rating Scale-Revised.*

The Parent Rating Scales measure a child's adaptive and challenging behaviors in the home and community settings. It is written in fourth-grade reading level. The reliabilities of the individual scales are high, with median values ranging from 0.80 to 0.87 at child and adolescent levels. The median test-retest reliability (7–90 days) of individual scales ranges 0.84 and 0.81 for child and adolescent levels, respectively. Median interrater reliabilities are 0.90 and 0.77 for child and adolescent levels, respectively. The correlations with Conners' Parent Rating scale are moderate to high (Kamphaus & Reynolds, 2004).

The Self-Report of Personality (SRP) is an "omnibus personality inventory" (Reynolds & Kamphaus, 2004, p. 4). SRP is written at a third grade reading level. The internal consistencies of the individual scales are high, with median values near 0.80. Median values of test-retest reliability of the individual scales are 0.75 and 0.84 at child and adolescent levels. The correlations with CBCL Youth Self-Report are moderate to high.

Since children with EOS usually present with multiple diagnoses and emotional/behavioral disturbances over the course of their illness, several of the primary scale scores may be elevated on the BASC-II. On the PRS and TRS, there are two scales that uniquely provide information about the child's functioning – Atypicality and Withdrawal. Assuming that the validity indexes are acceptable, it is important to conduct an item analysis that critically examines these scales. For example, on the Atypicality scale, school psychologists can examine items that would indicate positive symptoms, such as being out touch with reality or hearing or seeing things that are not there. Other items will indicate if they have strange ideas or are unable to block out unwanted thoughts. The Withdrawal scale may also reflect negative symptoms and social difficulties, such as avoiding peers, having difficulty making friends, or refusing to join others. On the SPR, item analysis, particularly on the Atypicality scale, can also indicate symptoms such as auditory or visual hallucinations and paranoia.

Personality Inventory for Youth (PIY; Lachar & Gruber, 1995). This measure is an objective multidimensional test of child and adolescent (9–19 years of age) behavior and emotional adjustment, family interaction, and neuro-cognitive and attention-related academic functioning. It contains 270 items that are completed by the child's parent or other rater who knows the child well. It takes about 45 minutes to complete. The *PIY* has adequate response validity check which makes it useful in ruling out psychiatric problems. *PIY* yields 10 clinical scales and 24 subscales measuring distinct and nonoverlapping clinical symptoms. The 10 clinical scales are Cognitive Impairment, Impulsivity/Distractibility, Delinquency, Family Dysfunction, Reality Distortion, Somatic Concern, Psychological Dysfunction, Social Withdrawal, Social Skill Deficits, and Classroom Screening Scale. There are also four validity scales which help determine if a respondent completes the items in a cooperative, careful, and honest manner or if he or she fully understands an item. Discriminant, convergent, and predictive validities have been established (Kline, Lachar & Sprague, 1985).

The three instruments described above – *CBCL*, *BASC-II*, and *PIY* – have been widely used by school psychologists as part of a comprehensive battery to diagnose students with potential ADHD, conduct problems, emotional disturbances, or autism. As described in the earlier sections of this chapter, these problems may also be warning signs of EOS. Therefore, information obtained from these assessment instruments may compliment other instruments in the diagnostic process.

Children's Global Assessment Scale (CGAS; Shaffer et al., 1983). Adapted from the Global Assessment Scale (GAS), *CGAS* is designed to reflect a child's level of functioning during a specified time period. The values of *CGAS* range from 1 to100, with 1 representing the lowest functioning level, 100 the highest, and 70 indicating normal function. Behaviorally oriented descriptors are presented at each anchor point, and they are used to describe behaviors and life situations applicable to children 4–16 years of age. Test-retest reliability (6 month) was 0.86, and interrater reliability was 0.84. Concurrent validity with Conner's Index was – 0.25. *CGAS* measures a child's overall functioning. Individuals with a 30% drop of functioning in comparison with the result obtained a year ago and with a psychotic illness in a first-or second-degree relative are considered at risk or prodromal for schizophrenia spectrum disorders.

*Brief Psychiatric Rating Scale for Children (*BPRS-C; Mullins, Pfefferbaum, Schultz & Overall, 1986; Lachar et al., 2001). *BPRS-C* is a 21-item, clinician-based rating scale designed to evaluate psychiatric problems among children and adolescents (Table 5.3). The *BPRS-C* yields seven relatively independent factors represented by three items each and a total score. The seven scales are: Behavior Problems, Depression, Thinking Disturbance, Psychomotor Excitation, Withdrawal

Table 5.3 Brief Psychiatric Rating Scale-Children (With Permission from Wolters Kluwer/ Lippincott Williams & Wilkins)

Items (definition)	Subscales (item number)
1. Uncooperativeness (negative, uncooperative, resistant, difficult to manage)	Behavior problems (1, 2, 3)
2. Hostility (angry or suspicious affect, belligerence, accusations and verbal condemnations of others)	
3. Manipulativeness (lying, cheating, exploitive of others)	
4. Depressed mood (sad, tearful, depressive demeanor)	Depression (4, 5, 6)
5. Feelings of inferiority (lacking self confidence, self-depreciatory, feeling of personal inadequacy)	
6. Suicidal ideation (thoughts, threats, or attempts of suicide)	
7. Peculiar fantasies (recurrent, odd, unusual, or autistic ideations)	Thought disturbance (7, 8, 9)
8. Delusions (ideas of reference, persecutory or grandiose delusions)	
9. Hallucinations (visual, auditory, or other hallucinatory experiences or perceptions)	
10. Hyperactivity (excessive energy expenditure, frequent changes in posture, perpetual motion)	Psychomotor excitation (10, 11,12)
11. Distractibility (poor concentration, shortened attention span, reactivity to peripheral stimuli)	
12. Speech or voice pressure (loud, excessive or pressured speech)	
13. Underproductive speech (minimal, spares inhibited verbal response pattern, or weak low voice)	Withdrawal-retardation (13, 14, 15)
14. Emotional withdrawal (unspontaneous relations to examiner, lack of peer interaction)	
15. Blunted affect (deficient emotional expression, blankness, flatness of affect)	
16. Tension (nervousness, fidgetiness, nervous movements of hands or feet)	Anxiety (16, 17, 18)
17. Anxiety (cling behavior, separation anxiety, preoccupation with anxiety topics, fears or phobias)	
18. Sleeping difficulties (inability to fall asleep, intermittent awakening, shortened sleep time)	
19. Disorientation (confusion over persons, places or things)	Organicity (19, 20, 21)
20. Speech deviance (inferior level of speech development, underdeveloped vocabulary, mispronunciation)	
21. Stereotype (rhythmic, repetitive, manneristic movements or posture)	

Ratings of each BPRS-C item are based on a 7-point Likert scale (not present, very mild, mild, moderate, moderately severe, severe, or extremely severe). Scores of each subscale range from 3 to 21. An individual is considered as having significant psychotic symptoms if he or she has a score of at least moderate on at least one of the key positive psychotic items (Items 7, 8, 9).

Retardation, Anxiety, and Organicity. Lachar et al. (2001) examined the reliability and reliability of an anchored version of BPRS-C. This anchored version contains a definition of the domain for each item and examples of behaviors. At item level, participants with a psychotic diagnosis scored lower on hyperactivity and higher on 10 of the 21 items – depressed mood, suicidal ideation, peculiar fantasies, delusions, hallucinations, underproductive speech, emotional withdrawal, blunted affect, anxiety, and sleep difficulties. At the scale level, the participants were rated as more depressed, showing more severe symptoms of thought disturbance, anxiety, withdrawal-retardation, internalization, developmental maladjustment, and total pathology. The internal consistency was adequate for the total score and six of the seven subscale scores (>0.69), except the anxiety scale with a coefficient alpha of 0.57. Interrater reliability coefficients range from 0.75 to 0.91. Concurrent validity has been established in that the rating scores of BPRS-C scales were consistent with the diagnosis of the participants.

The *BPRS-C* is an efficient way to document the complete symptoms. It complements clinician ratings of functional impairment as measured by scales like CGAS. The administration time is about 20–30 min, in the context of a clinical interview with the child and the parent(s).

Interview. The *Schedule for Affective Disorders and Schizophrenia for School-Age Children – Present and lifetime Version* (K-SADS-PL; Kaufman et al., 1997; Kaufman, Birmaher, Brent, Rao, & Ryan, 1996). The *K-SADS-PL* assesses both lifetime and current psychiatric diagnoses. There are six sections in *K-SADS-PL*: (a) an unstructured Introductory Interview; (b) a Diagnostic Screening Interview; (c) the Supplement Completion Checklist; (d) the appropriate Diagnostic Supplements; (e) the Summary Lifetime Diagnoses Checklist; and f) the Children's Global Assessment Scale (C-GAS) ratings. The first four sections are completed with each informant separately; the last two sections are completed after synthesizing all the data and resolving discrepancies in informants' reports.

The Introductory Interview is used to establish rapport. The Diagnostic Screening Interview consists of 82 symptom items which form 20 diagnostic areas. If a child receives even one threshold rating (3 – "definitely present"), he or she will be administered one or more of the six diagnostic disorders on the Diagnostic Supplements, which include Affective Disorders, Psychotic Disorders, Anxiety Disorders, Behavioral Disorders, Substance Use, and Other Disorders. The Summary Lifetime Diagnoses Checklist summarizes lifetime diagnostic information based on the synthesis of the data from all sources. Lastly, C-GAS is used to examine the existence of functional decline. The interrater agreement of the Diagnostic Supplement scales range from 93–100%, and test–retest reliability estimates were adequate. Concurrent validity of the supplement scales has also been established. Specifically, children who met the criteria of depression or anxiety also scored significantly higher children on the CBCL internalizing scales. The *K-SADS-PL* provides diagnosis-specific impairment ratings to assist diagnostic determination.

NIMH Diagnostic Interview Schedule for Children (NIMH-DISC; Shaffer, Fisher, Lucas, Dulcan, & Schwab-Stone, 2000). The *NIMH DISC* is a structured psychiatric diagnostic interview for children and adolescents aged 6–18 and their parents. There are parallel versions of the instrument: the DISC-P for parents (or knowledgeable caretakers) of 6–17-year-olds, and the DISC-Y (for direct administration to children and youths aged 9–17 years of age). The most recent revision of the DISC (NIMH DISC-IV) is based on *DSM-IV* diagnostic criteria. The *NIMH DISC* can be administered by trained lay interviewers who are instructed to administer the queries exactly as written. The schizophrenia section of the Diagnostic Interview Schedule for Children is composed of five questions regarding possible psychotic symptoms which were scored as no (0); yes, likely (1); and yes, definitely (2). In clinical settings, the *NIMH DISC* can serve as a diagnostic aid, freeing the clinician from making lengthy inquiries about the symptoms. However, it cannot address invalid responses given by a respondent who misunderstands a question and it does not allow unusual presentations, being restricted to assessing symptoms in the *DSM* systems. As with other instruments, the *NIMH DISC* should be used as one of the instruments in a comprehensive assessment battery and it cannot replace usual clinical practice.

Positive and Negative Syndrome Scale for Children (Kiddie-PANSS; Fields et al., 1994). The Kiddie-PANSS is designed to identify and interpret schizophrenia symptoms. There are 30 operationalized symptom items in the *Kiddie-PANSS* (together with specific criteria for severity levels), which yield seven positive symptoms (hallucinatory behavior, delusions, disorganized speech, etc.), as well as seven negative symptoms (poor rapport, emotional withdrawal, blunted affect, etc.). It also has 16 items that make up the general psychopathology scale, which is used as a measure of control for overall psychopathology. The *Kiddie-PANSS* includes one semistructured, prepatient interview with the primary caregiver and one interview with the patient (both semistructured and structured). A structured play interview is used with younger children (6–10 years of age) to accommodate their language ability. Interrater correlations of the three subscales (positive syndrome, negative syndrome, and general psychopathology) and total psychopathology range from 0.76 to 0.86. The *Kiddie-PANSS* scores are highly correlated with the *DSM-III-R* diagnosis of schizophrenia, but not with Achenbach's *CBCL* subscales.

Direct Assessment

Direct observational methods involve the observation of the target behavior(s) at the moment when the behavior is occurring (Li, 2004). These methods employ direct observation of an individual's overt behavior such as motoric movements, speech, facial expression, tone of voice, groom and hygiene or reaction to the environment in either naturalistic (e.g., school or home) or analogue settings (clinic or hospital). Moreover, direct observational methods (except the self-monitoring procedure) use an independent person to observe and report on an individual's overt behaviors.

Unlike the assessment of autism or ADHD, there is a lack of standardized direct assessment instruments of EOS. However, school psychologists are trained to make clinical observations when evaluating a student. Further, parents and school teachers observe a child or youth on daily basis; their input is crucial in establishing an accurate diagnosis. In addition to the aforementioned behaviors that are observable to a school psychologist during the psychological assessment, *BPRS* and *K-SADS-PL* have sections that may guide direct assessment of an individual's school and home behaviors. For example, teachers may observe a student at risk of developing EOS as being absent more from school than before, being more disruptive in class, staying alone during recess, and having poorer academic performance (e.g., from a B student to a C or failing student). Parents may complain that the child has gradually or abruptly stopped talking to them or his/her siblings, and he/she cannot fall asleep at night, walking aimlessly inside or around the house, and less attentive to hygiene. People who live or work with the child may notice that he/she talks strangely, using odd phrases or words or talking in circles and rambling, or being incoherent when expressing himself or herself. More severely, a child or youth may be seen talking to themselves excessively or becoming violent toward self or others. Some youth with EOS may be seen "bragging" that they have superpower to cure people or turning to look at, smell, or touch things when there is no one or nothing near them. Mental health professionals, teachers, and parents may also see a child being sad or angry more easily, having difficulty initiating and finishing work, lack of energy, day dreaming, or easily getting upset even under normal stress.

The aforementioned observations of a child's symptoms may be indicative of different problems and they are useful in informing diagnosis of EOS. It should be noted that some observations of a child's behavior may not match between or among observers. This is expected as the child is observed at different settings, at different events, and at different times of the day. The observations complement each other. When there is great variability in the observations, a functional behavioral assessment that monitors symptom presentation, identifies circumstances and settings that are highly problematic for the child, and engages multiple stakeholders can create a comprehensive picture of the child's functioning.

Concluding Comments

EOS is a complicated and debilitating developmental neurological disorder. It is essential that school psychologists who work with children and adolescents on a daily basis know its symptoms, diagnostic criteria, developmental and clinical course, associated syndromes, and assessment instruments and procedures. Such knowledge will help school psychologists and other education professionals to identify early warning signs of the illness, make timely referral to child psychiatrists, and provide clinical information to other mental health professionals to reach an accurate diagnosis, thus enabling an effective treatment process.

Chapter 6
Psychoeducational Assessment

Students presenting with complex patterns of emotional and behavioral difficulties occur with a degree of frequency in school settings – particularly in light of the Surgeon General's Report on Mental Health (US Department of Health and Human Services, 1999) which indicated that approximately 20% of children and adolescents demonstrate symptoms qualifying them for diagnoses under the *Diagnostic and Statistical Manual of Mental Disorders – Fourth Edition* (DSM-IV; APA, 2000). For a student to be diagnosed with early onset schizophrenia (EOS), s/he must demonstrate a degree of functional impairment; thus, the school psychologist may already be aware of the needs of the student. This is particularly true if the student is in an active phase of the illness with ongoing delusions and hallucinations. It is not necessarily the responsibility of school personnel to make the diagnosis of EOS, yet all school psychologists should be able to conduct the psychoeducational evaluation of students with schizophrenia and other psychotic spectrum disorders.

As mentioned in previous chapters, the diagnostic criteria outlined in the (DSM-IV) (APA, 2000) are not synonymous with the *Individuals with Disabilities Education Improvement Act* (IDEIA, 2004) eligibility criteria. Special education law clearly stipulates that having a disability alone does not warrant eligibility for special education services and requires that the disability must impact the child's ability to make effective academic progress. Even though the federal definition of "emotional disturbance" specifically indicates that this category includes "students who are schizophrenic," youth with high premorbid functioning may still function adequately academically, especially with appropriate pharmacological and psychosocial treatment. For example, in a multisite national study of children and adolescents with EOS, 51% continued to be educated in the regular education setting and roughly one-third were educated in resource rooms or self-contained special education classrooms (Frazier et al., 2007).

Consequently, the differences in diagnostic and educational eligibility criteria highlight the need for school psychologists to conduct their own psychoeducational assessments to create a profile of the student's social, behavioral, and academic strengths and weaknesses, which can serve as a foundation for creating education and treatment plans as well as monitoring overall functioning in the school setting. The information gathered from a psychoeducational evaluation can assist school

H. Li et al., *Identifying, Assessing, and Treating Early Onset Schizophrenia at School*, Developmental Psychopathology at School, DOI 10.1007/978-1-4419-6272-0_6,

personnel as they meet the unique educational needs of the student with EOS. Many students with EOS need support services (e.g., 504 accommodations or *IDEIA* special education services) for successful educational experiences (Frazier et al., 2007), though these services need to be determined on a case-by-case basis by each education team based, in large part, on the psychoeducational evaluation conducted by the school psychologist.

There are considerations to make when planning a psychoeducational evaluation of students with EOS, such as their current level of functioning or impairment, developmental level, and the phase of their illness. For example, knowing the developmental level of a student becomes critical when conducting an evaluation of a student experiencing ongoing period of psychosis. Symptoms that are normal at younger ages, such as imaginary friends, would be considered psychotic in late adolescence or adulthood (Kronenberger & Meyer, 2001). As such, when conducting a psychoeducational evaluation with students with EOS, the challenge is in determining whether the obtained scores reflect their skills and abilities or the psychological impairments due to the mental illness.

The social, behavioral, and cognitive deficits associated with EOS can require modification and accommodation of assessment practices to obtain the most accurate representation of the students' current level of performance. This chapter focuses on issues unique to conducting a psychoeducational assessment with students at the prodromal stage or students with EOS and offers strategies to obtain the most accurate representation of their skills and abilities. The following sections of this chapter provide a review of testing accommodations and modifications that may be necessary to obtain valid results, and then a review of specific psychoeducational assessment findings and practices.

Testing Considerations, Accommodations, and Modifications

When conducting a psychoeducational assessment with a student with EOS, the school psychologist may or may not initially be aware of overt psychopathology. The student may be functioning adequately in the school environment, based on the current phase of illness and/or treatment efficacy, yet subtle signs may become more apparent over the course of the evaluation. The two primary characteristics of schizophrenia – positive symptoms and negative symptoms – may become more noticeable when using standardized assessment tools and the student begins demonstrating peculiar or bizarre response patterns. Each student demonstrating psychotic symptoms or having EOS will have their own individual and unique presentation; therefore, there is no single set of accommodations that will work for every student. In this context, the examiners must do their best to follow best practices and standardization procedures while also being flexible with these practices in order to obtain the most accurate results. Recommendations and strategies to accomplish these goals are discussed below.

Considerations Based on the Subtype

Schizophrenia is not a unidimensional diagnosis and the various subtypes – paranoid, catatonic, disorganized, undifferentiated, residual – can present very differently in a psychoeducational evaluation. For example, a student with the paranoid type of EOS may demonstrate adequate cognitive functioning and lack disorganized speech or inappropriate affect, but demonstrate prominent delusions or auditory hallucinations of a persecutory or grandiose nature (APA, 2000). In contrast, a student with the disorganized type of EOS may present with disorganized speech, total incoherence, neologisms (nonsense words), or echolalia accompanied by physically disorganized behavior such as repetitive purposeless activity, odd posturing, or disruption in the ability to perform activities of daily living, such as showering or dressing (APA, 2000).

When planning the psychoeducational evaluation, it can be helpful to have as much information about the EOS psychiatric diagnosis and subtype to plan for the necessary modifications and accommodations. For example, when assessing students with gross and pervasive disorganization, it can be helpful to start with tasks that have strict standardization procedures and are highly structured (e.g., cognitive and achievement testing). These students may have difficulty engaging in verbally-laden tasks, thus requiring the assessment to focus on nonverbal processing skills. Students who are paranoid, however, might need to be given choices on the organization of the tasks with constant transparency about the process. For example, it could be disturbing for a student with paranoia to have an examiner sit with a clipboard taking notes. Rather, the examiner can share with the student the activities that need to be accomplished, the notes and information being recorded, and frequent updates on the assessment process. For those with catatonic inhibition (e.g., decreased activity level, limited speech), the examiner may need to provide opportunities for the students to communicate in writing or by drawing the responses. In all of these examples, behavioral observations and copious notes are critical components of the evaluation as they document the modifications of standardized procedures necessary for completion of the assessment.

Considerations Based on the Phase

The phase of the illness (active, recovery, residual) is also important to consider when designing a psychoeducational evaluation of a student with EOS. Students who are in the recovery or residual phase of their illness may be able to provide accurate information about their history, current experiences, and treatment. They may also be able to discuss the challenges they are experiencing in the school setting, thus requiring few or no specific modifications or accommodations. If they are in the active phase, however, they may not be able to provide accurate information and the evaluation will need to be greatly modified to obtain their mental status (Fontaine, 2009). In these cases, the school will instead need to assist the caregivers as they obtain medical and psychiatric evaluations to ascertain the student's level of safety while also creating an intervention plan.

Communicate with Caregivers and/or Medical Providers

A student who has a diagnosis of EOS may be closely monitored by other health care providers, such as psychiatrists. Communicating with health care providers and caregivers *prior* to conducting the psychoeducational evaluation is a critical component of obtaining the best performance from the student. Recent changes in medications or symptoms indicative of a decline in functioning can compromise the accuracy of the information being gathered for the evaluation. If there are significant concerns about the stability of the student's emotional state or phase of illness, then the educational evaluation team may need to reconvene to alter timelines that meet the legal mandates *and* accurately represent the child's current level of functioning. For example, one of the authors was conducting a cognitive assessment as part of a triennial re-evaluation with a female student demonstrating severe decompensation (e.g., hallucinations, decline in hygiene, affective, and behavioral instability). The first few subtests were indicating very low cognitive abilities, which were not commensurate with previous observations of the student's academic and cognitive functioning. The parents and the education team met, based on these preliminary findings and behavioral observations, and ultimately the student had a brief psychiatric hospitalization where medications were altered and she was stabilized. The parents agreed, in writing, to extend the mandated timelines so that a more accurate representation of her abilities could be determined when she was more stable. The cognitive assessment continued with a re-administration of the ceiling items of the first few subtests and completion of the remaining portions of the test. The first administration, based on a prorated analysis, would have indicated cognitive abilities in the deficient range, but after the student stabilized the scores indicated low average scores.

Parents and caregivers will want evaluations completed in a timely manner, but their larger concern may be with having an accurate representation of their child's functioning and abilities. Conducting evaluations during periods of heightened stress or during periods of compromised reality testing can result in inaccurate findings, and these findings can follow the student for the rest of their life. As in the example above, if educational planning was determined based on the initial findings, this student may have been inappropriately placed; thus highlighting the need for best efforts to accurately assess students with EOS. Inaccurate assessment results can cause indeterminable harm to the student and should be avoided when possible.

Preparing the Student for the Evaluation

For a student recently diagnosed or one who has never engaged in a psychoeducational evaluation, he or she may have difficulty adjusting to changes in his or her daily routine that will be required as part of completing the assessment. To reduce the stress associated with novel situations, the student can have specific time blocked out of his or her daily schedule over a period of time while he or she becomes familiar with the examiner, testing room, and testing experience. It can also help to have a few meetings with the student in the testing room prior to any formal evaluation being conducted.

By the time the student has already received the EOS diagnosis, however, he or she may have participated in many evaluations with medical and educational personnel. It can be helpful to find out from other professionals and caregivers about any recent evaluations conducted in clinical or medical settings to reduce the risk of re-administration of the same tests. For those students, the school psychologist may need to conduct his or her own evaluation to ascertain the students' current capacity to process tasks and manage the stress of the school environment. These students may only need a reminder of what the assessment entails and how the information will be used. If the student has recently participated in testing, then it is essential to work with parents or caregivers, obtaining written approval to review his or her assessment strategies, results, and recommendations.

Specific Psychoeducational Assessment Practices

Just as it is critically important to demonstrate necessary modifications and accommodations to complete a psychoeducational evaluation with a student with EOS, it is also crucial to be knowledgeable of appropriate assessment practices and tools. This section reviews the types of information, such as behavioral observation, file reviews, and interviews that assist with educational planning, as well as specific areas of functioning (e.g., cognitive, adaptive behavior, language funsctioning, psychological processes, and academic development) that need to be evaluated for students with EOS.

Behavioral Observation, Functional Assessment, and Interviews

Behavioral observations are essential components of a comprehensive evaluation to ascertain functional impairment due to EOS (Kodish & McClellan, 2007). Because the illness is dynamic, it is important to obtain multiple data points, especially when the EOS is emerging or in various phases (Wozniak, White, & Schulz, 2005). These observations can determine functional abilities in a variety of settings, serve as a foundation for educational planning, and assist the school psychologists as they plan the psychoeducational evaluation.

Observations conducted in a variety of classes can identify academic areas that are challenging as well as social situations that result in behavioral dysfunction. As an example, a student with EOS may perform adequately in a lecture-based course, such as a math class, where there are minimal social interactions and clear, straight forward answers. However, the student may present with more problems in a class such as health, where there are frequent class discussions that focus on areas of personal difficulty for the student (e.g., hygiene, self-care social relationships), or even language arts, where fiction literature or creative writing tasks that could trigger thought distortions or even disorganized speech. Observations of unstructured occasions, such as lunch or class transition time, provide information of potentially stressful or taxing social situations that can negatively impact educational performance and interpersonal relationships. Systematic, time sampling observations methods, with tools such as the *Systematic Observation System* of the *Behavior Assessment System for Children – Second Edition,* (Reynolds & Kamphaus, 2004), may provide useful information during active phases of illness, yet may not adequately capture low incidence behaviors associated with EOS.

Information gathered from academic and social observations can serve as the foundation for a functional analysis of behavioral difficulties, thus leading to targeted interventions that meet the unique needs of the student. For example, a student with EOS may consistently skip the class that occurs after lunch. This may reflect the stress the student experiences in minimally supervised, socially pressured situations, and simple strategies such as eating lunch in a quiet location with a small, supportive peer group can increase the student's success in the school day. Targeted interventions derived from a functional behavioral assessment can be the basis for creating successful school experiences for students with EOS. More information about functional behavioral assessments can be found in Table 6.1 as well as in resource materials such as O'Neill et al. (1997) book listed in the references.

Interviews with multiple stakeholders also provide information that builds on the observations and assessment results, particularly when targeting strengths and weaknesses for the student with EOS. Interviews with parents and caregivers can provide information about the medical, social, and educational development of the child; areas of strength and vulnerability; and challenges at home, school, and community settings. They will have information on how the student engages socially with other family members and in the community as well as situations where the student experiences success and challenges. They may share the student's perceptions of teachers and classes where the student achieves and where s/he struggles. They will know the student's coping strategies that can be integrated into educational planning for the school.

Table 6.1 Key Components of a Functional Behavior Assessment

1. A clear description of the problem behaviors in measurable, observable terms
2. Identification of the events, times, situations that attempt to predict when the problem behaviors *will* and *will not* occur
3. Identification of the consequences that maintain the problem behaviors (the function/reason)
4. Development of one or more summary statements or hypotheses that describe the behavior and its functions
5. Collection of direct observation data

Drasgow & Yell (2001): Copyright 2001 by the National Association of School Psychologists, Bethesda, MD. Reprinted with permission of the publisher, www.nasponline.org

Within the school setting, teachers will have information about how the student functions in the classroom setting – both socially and academically. Information from other school personnel, such as cafeteria or custodial staff, can also identify situations in the school day that may need to be addressed. School administrators will have information on discipline or attendance issues for the student. Finally, gathering information from the school nurse is imperative as s/he may have knowledge about medication management, physical manifestations of stress, and overall physical and mental health status.

Comprehensive File Review

A thorough review of school records is an informative assessment tool, especially since it can provide information on a pattern of functioning, which may reflect a decline due to the illness (Kodish & McClellan, 2008). School records contain an enormous amount of information regarding historical trends, such as patterns or reasons of difficulty, attendance, social relations, academic performance, and effort. By reviewing developmental screenings, such as entry to kindergarten, or annual academic testing, the school psychologist can identify cognitive and academic functioning as well as changes over their school experiences. If available, medical records can establish developmental and social history, if not already available in school records. As previously mentioned, these records may also indicate previous testing in clinical setting. These assessments may have been conducted during periods of heightened stress (e.g., during a psychiatric inpatient hospitalization) and can provide data on the functional capacity of the student in various phases of the illness.

Psychoeducational Testing

In addition to the diagnostic evaluation data mentioned in Chapter 5, a number of psychoeducational measures are appropriate when ascertaining the student's present levels of functioning, particularly as it relates to school performance. The following measures are assessment tools that can be included in the psychoeducational evaluations of a student with EOS.

Cognitive functioning. Consistent with the adult literature, low intellectual functioning is associated with EOS. Lower IQ "may reflect a causal factor for the psychotic manifestations of schizophrenia, predisposing an individual to the development of false beliefs and perceptions" (Lewis & Levitt, 2002, p. 418). Cognitive delays were once thought to be a "consequence" of the schizophrenia, but it is now believed to be a potential precursor or general risk to psychopathology and a sign of vulnerability to the illness (McClellan & Werry, 2001; Wozniak et al., 2005).

A meta-analytic study was conducted by Woodberry, Giuliano, and Seidman (2008), which examined 18 studies comparing the IQs of individuals assessed premorbid and after receiving the diagnosis of schizophrenia, primarily as adults. The authors concluded that those who develop schizophrenia have a modest deficit in global cognition, with the subjects demonstrating an average IQ of 94.7. These findings were consistent whether the intelligence testing was done with comprehensive tools (e.g., Wechsler system) or group-administered tools (e.g., Draft Board Tests). There were also no significant differences between verbal and nonverbal domains, no differences between genders, and no definitive evidence of decline in IQ with age during the premorbid period.

For those with EOS, other studies have also supported the findings of more global IQ deficits using the *Wechsler Intelligence Scale for Children* (2003), with full scale IQs (FSIQ) in the low average range, that may be evident before the onset of symptoms (Fagerlund, Pagsberg, & Hemmingsen, 2006; Frazier et al., 2007; Wozniak et al., 2005). Similar to adult literature, those with EOS demonstrated an initial steep decline in IQ in the period between about 2 years prior to the first psychotic episode and 2 years after diagnosis. More specifically, the average pre-onset FSIQ scores for this group dropped 10 points from the low average range (90) to below average/borderline range (80) in the post-onset period (Gochman et al., 2005).

Intellectual impairment does not classify a subgroup of individuals with schizophrenia; however, at least 10–20% of children with EOS have IQs in the borderline to mentally retarded range (Asarnow & Ben-Meir, 1988; Davidson et al., 1999; Kenny et al., 1997). Overall, the association of low IQ and EOS is very modest (3% of cases of schizophrenia; Lewis & Levitt, 2002). Assessing cognitive functioning as one aspect of a psychoeducational evaluation can determine the degree of impairment associated with the illness and help guide education and treatment planning.

In addition to the cognitive impairments, suggesting widespread brain dysfunction, there are consistent reports of specific neuropsychological deficits in individuals with schizophrenia – including those with EOS (Cervellion, Burdick, Cottone, Rhinewine, & Kumra, 2007; Seidman et al., 2006). Impairments in secondary memory (e.g., verbal learning and memory functions) have been associated with an earlier onset of schizophrenia. Secondary memory, which is assessed with tools such as the *California Verbal Learning Test* (CVLT: Delis, Krammer, Kaplan, and Ober, 1987), is the "ability to the ability to acquire and store information over a longer period of time (usually lasting for several minutes and longer)" and "exceeds the immediate memory span" (Green, Kern, Braff, & Mintz, 2000, p. 127). In their epidemiological study, Tuulio-Henriksson Partonen, Suvisaari, Haukka, and Lonnqvist (2004) concluded that "verbal learning and memory functions may be particularly vulnerable to the developmental process leading to schizophrenia" as well as "undermine the social adaptation and educational possibilities" (p. 218). Additionally, Rhinewine et al. (2005) reported no significant differences in the neurocognitive profiles of those with childhood- and adolescent-onset, yet those who experience multiple episodes of psychosis experience more deficits in functioning than those experiencing one episode. Individuals who experienced psychosis were equally impaired in the areas of attention and spatial memory; however, those with multiple episodes were significantly more impaired in the areas of executive functioning, psychomotor speed, and pattern memory (Braw et al., 2008).

A meta-analytic study by Green et al. (2000) related neurocognitive deficits to functional outcomes in adult populations. Secondary memory impairments were related to functional impairments in every outcome domain – Community/ Daily activities, Social problem solving, and Psychosocial skill acquisition. Impairment in immediate verbal memory, or "the ability to hold a limited amount of information for a brief period of time" (p. 127), was linked to impairment in acquisition of psychosocial skills. Cervellione et al. (2007) demonstrated similar links between neurocognitive deficits and functional impairment in adolescents with EOS. The adolescents were impaired in attention/vigilance and working memory, which were significantly related to decreased social and communication, personal and community living skills. Furthermore, they found that attention and vigilance was significantly associated with personal and community living skills and working memory was associated with personal living skills.

Academic/developmental functioning. The school psychologist may or may not conduct the academic assessment; however, it may be necessary to assist other psychoeducational assessment team members to identify strategies that obtain the most accurate representation of the student's functioning. This is a critical issue because inaccurate findings can misrepresent the student's skills and lead to flawed educational plans, which is a serious concern since the educational outcomes of students with emotional disturbance continue to be the worst of any disability group, despite being an educational priority of the federal department of education since the mid-1960s (Bradley, Henderson, & Monfore, 2004). To date, very few studies have examined the academic functioning of students with EOS (Wozniak et al., 2005). For example, the multisite study of children with EOS (Frazier et al. 2007) reported limited academic information about the subjects, offering only that more than a quarter had repeated a grade. In addition, a recent national cohort study completed in Sweden indicated that poor school performance and failing classes were significantly associated with an increased risk for schizophrenia (MacCabe et al., 2008).

The most comprehensive study of academic assessment was completed by Fuller et al. (2002), which examined the retrospective group academic assessment (Iowa Test of Basic Skills) data for 70 adults with schizophrenia. The subjects' performance, based on state percentile ranks, was analyzed for grades 4, 8, and 11 in the areas of vocabulary, reading comprehension, language, mathematics, sources of information (reading diagrams and charts), and composite scores. The results indicated that those who went on to develop schizophrenia fell below the state norms on every category for all three grades, although there were no significant differences at the fourth or eighth grade assessment for any categories. By the 11th grade, however, scores were significantly lower than peers in the areas of reading, language, sources of information, and composite. Moreover, the language scores became progressively worse from grade 4, 8, and 11. The authors suggest that this decline between the eighth and 11th grade – or ages 13 and 16, the onset of puberty – may be a precursor to the cognitive impairment that accompanies the first psychotic episode. Additionally, the mean age of this study was 28 years, yet there were no differences between those with illness onset prior to age 20 and those with the onset at age 20 or later. These findings suggest that more research and information is needed on the impact of EOS on academic development.

Accurate assessments serve as the foundation to creating the best educational opportunities for students with EOS. Academic functioning can be assessed with state-of-the-art tools such as the *Woodcock-Johnson III Tests of Achievement* (WJ III – Ach; Woodcock, McGrew, & Mather, 2001) and *Wechsler Individual Achievement Tests – Third Edition* (WIAT-III; Wechsler, 2009). These comprehensive assessment tools organize subtests into cluster and domain scores in the areas of reading, mathematics, and written and oral language. In addition to the findings from the individually administered assessment tools, it can be helpful to contextualize the student's performance by examining results from group administered achievement tests. These assessment tools, however, may not adequately reflect academic performance in the classroom setting, therefore other measures, such as curriculum based assessments, homework completion, and class attendance, also need to be closely examined.

Adaptive behavior. The domains assessed in adaptive scales – motor, communication, socialization, and daily living skills – will frequently be deficient for those with EOS, particularly given the nature of this disorder (Kronenberger & Meyer, 2001). The deficiencies in adaptive behavior will vary by subtype, but global deficits have been demonstrated in those identified with schizophrenia while young. For example, using the *Vineland Adaptive Behavior Scale* (VABS; Sparrow, Balla, & Cichetti, 1984), Frazier et al. (2007) found significant deficits in overall adaptive behavior, with an average score less than 60, or more than two standard deviations below the mean.

Over the past two decades, there has been increasing evidence of neuromotor abnormalities preceding the onset of schizophrenia (Fish et al., 1992; Hans & Marcus 1991; Walker & Lewine, 1990). The British birth cohort studies found both speech and motor difficulties in infancy and speech and word pronunciation problems at age 7 and 11 years to be predictive of later onset of schizophrenia. Infant offspring of parents with schizophrenia have been found to show developmental delays in motor functions. Similarly, child and adolescent offspring of schizophrenia parents manifest greater deficits than children of normal and affective-disordered parents on measures of motor proficiency and neurologic soft signs (e.g., poor motor coordination, sensory perceptual difficulties, and difficulties in sequencing of complex motor tasks). Using the archival video observational approach to analyzing motor behaviors of infants who later developed schizophrenia, Walker and Lewine (1990) found limb posture and movement abnormalities and a trend toward hypotonicity in the preschizophrenia infants, though such dysfunction is not unique to schizophrenia. They also found that the critical period from birth to 2 years was the only period during which there was a significant differentiation between those who later developed schizophrenia and those who did not. Basic human motor abilities, such as manual manipulation and locomotion, are in rapid development in the first 2 years; this may account for the group differences in motor skills during this critical period. Additionally, fine motor speed and dexterity deficits have been identified in those with EOS (Asarnow et al., 1994).

Language functioning. A speech and language pathologist should assess the student's language functioning whenever a student with EOS is being considered for special education services. The communication of many children who later developed schizophrenia is often referred to as odd or inappropriate. Developmental delays in speech and language production have been reported in individuals with COS and EOS and also in those who have a parent with schizophrenia (Hollis, 1995; Kolvin, Ounsted, Humphrey, & McNay, 1971). In fact, language impairment is found to be more common in EOS than in youth with other psychiatric illnesses (Fuller et al., 2002; Hollis, 1995). Studies have demonstrated that youth with EOS have more reading and spelling difficulties compared with normal controls, with males with EOS demonstrating more problems with speech development than females (Vourdas, Pipe, Corrigall, & Frangou, 2003). In some cases, children progressed from a long-standing communication disorder to the insidious onset of thought disorder and disorganized behavior which are hallmarks of EOS (Hollis, 1995). Semantic fluency, or the ability to verbally or nonverbally generate items belonging to a certain category of knowledge (e.g., animals, body parts) in a fixed time, is also seen as an early trait marker for those with EOS (Phillips, James, Crow, & Collinson, 2004). Furthermore, a longitudinal study of premorbid cognitive functioning in children who went on to develop schizophrenia showed a significant linear decline in language scores over time; with the authors suggesting that language impairments may be the first deficits to show in childhood, followed by more generalized cognitive and language impairments in teenage years (Fuller et al., 2002).

Emotional functioning. Impairments in emotional functioning are a marker of EOS. Chapter 5 discusses the diagnostic characteristics associated with this disorder as well as tools, such as the *Behavior Assessment System for Children – Second Edition* (BASC-2; Reynolds & Kamphaus, 2004) or the *Child Behavior Checklist* (CBCL; Achenbach & Rescorla, 2001) that assist with diagnostic interpretation and school-based interventions planning. As part of a psychoeducational evaluation, these assessment systems include rating forms that can gather information from teachers and school staff about the student's performance in multiple classroom environments and school activities. Therefore, it can be helpful to have various school personnel identify areas of strength and weakness of the student to assist with educational planning.

Studies that have used these assessment tools indicate significant impairment in emotional and behavioral functioning. In the multisite study by Frazier et al. (2007), the Total Problems score on Teacher rating scales from the *CBCL* were elevated ($t = 67$), and the Parent rating scales were significantly elevated ($t = 71$).

Table 6.2 Mental Status Exam

	Normal	Problem	Serious Problem
Appearance	Well-groomed Appropriate to season	Unkempt Unclean	Disorganized Disheveled Dirty Inappropriate to season
Posture	Comfortable Relaxed	Tense Limp	Rigid Slumped
Facial Expressions	Composed Engaged Interested	Anxious/ fearful Depression/ sadness Anger/ irritability	Staring/Dazed Limited expression Overt hostility Bizarre
Attitude	Cooperative Open	Detached Disengaged Guarded	Hostile Resistant Manipulative
Activity Level	Controlled Moderated	Hyperactive Lethargic	Catatonia Agitation Impulsive
Speech	Spontaneous Fluid	Slowed Increased/loud Decreased/ slowed	Poverty of speech Atypical quality Slurring/ Stammering
Pace	Modulated Rhythmic	Rapid Slow	Pressured/ Frenzied Monotone
Volume	Adequately audible	Loud Difficult to hear	Very loud/ Very soft Mute
Clarity	Intelligible	Unclear	Garbled Slurred
Content	Rational Logical Coherence	Loose associations Obscene	Rhyming /Clanging Neologisms Illogical rambling
Affect and Mood	Animated Congruent with content	Anxious /Sad Shameful Restricted Apathy	Euphoric/expansive Blunted/flat Dysphoric/depressed Labile/dramatic
Thought Content	Rational/ Logical Goal oriented	Preoccupations	Suicidal ideation* Homicidal ideation*
Perceptions	Grounded Aware	Delusions Intrusive thoughts or sensations	Active hallucinations* (auditory, visual, etc.) Bizarre delusions Paranoia Obsessions
Orientation	Person, Time, Place (x3)	Disoriented	Grossly disoriented Loss of awareness
Cognition/Memory	Short term memory Alert	Distractible Confused Inattentive	Unable to recall basic information

*Requires immediate assessment for safety and crisis planning in accordance with school policies and procedures.

The Youth Self-Report also reflected concerns ($t = 63$). Similar findings were reported by Patel et al. (2006) in their study comparing *CBCL* scores of children and adolescents with schizophrenia-spectrum disorders in three ethnic groups (African-American, Caucasian, and Hispanic). There were no significant differences in the Total Problems or Internalizing scores and all were significantly elevated (e.g., more than two standard deviations above the mean). However, there was a significant difference on the Externalizing score, with African-American and Caucasian students' scores in the at-risk range and Hispanic children demonstrating less externalizing behavioral difficulties, with scores in the average range.

For students with EOS, as a part of a comprehensive psychoeducational evaluation, it is important to assess the student's current mental status to get a baseline of psychological functioning. Observations of the student's verbal and nonverbal behavior, appearance, activity level, and attitude can serve as a foundation of this assessment. Their orientation to time and place as well as current events provides information about their thinking and cognitive organization. An example of a mental status exam, created by one of the authors, is in Table 6.2, and there are also commercial products available, such as the *Mental Status Checklist for Children* or the *Mental Status Checklist for Adolescents* (Dougherty & Schinka, 1989).

Finally, when students are actively experiencing hallucinations, it can be challenging to know the appropriate questions to ask. Examples of questions to gather necessary information are provided in Table 6.3. The information obtained from these questions can assist communications with other health care providers as they monitor the current status of the student as well as monitor treatment efficacy.

Summary

The findings from a psychoeducational assessment can illuminate the strengths and weakness of a student with EOS, thus leading to educational planning as well as life planning. The services and supports necessary for successful school experiences will vary for each student, and this evaluation is a critical component of the education planning. It is essential that school psychologists have basic competencies in assessing students with or at-risk of developing serious mental illness, such as psychosis and schizophrenia, and to identify concerns whether the student is referred for an initial or an ongoing evaluation. School professionals are in a unique position to identify problematic behaviors, and early identification and referrals to medical providers can alter the trajectory of the illness. The information gathered through a psychoeducational evaluation can assist with instructional planning and serve as a foundation for consulting with other school staff and professionals as they address the educational, behavioral, and social needs of the student with EOS.

Table 6.3 Interview Questions to Identify Hallucinations and Delusions

Hallucinations

Identify the senses impacted by the perceptual disturbance

- Did it seem like they were somewhere else, like outside of your head, or was it like a conversation inside your head?
- Would other people be able to hear this conversation?
- What did you hear/see/smell/touch/taste?
- Have you ever heard someone call your name when there was no one around, or hear music that other people could not?
- Has there ever been a time when you had an unusual smell about yourself?
- Has there ever been a time when you saw things that were not there?
- What about shadows or other objects moving? Did you ever see ghosts?
- Do the voices tell you to do anything? Or, do they tell you to hurt or kill yourself or someone else?

Ascertain a timeline and/or frequency of events

- When does this happen?
- Does it occur at night, while you were trying to sleep, or did it happen in the daytime too?
- Were you sick with fever when they occurred?
- Were you drinking beer/liquor or taking any drugs when it happened?
- Did it last for several days or several times a week?

Get a sense of their reaction to these experiences

- Did you think it was real when you (heard, saw, etc.) it, or did you think it was your imagination?
- What did you do when you (heard, saw, etc.) it?

Consider Cultural /diversity issues

- Do other people in your family or church have similar experiences?

Delusions

General questions to gather information on nature of delusions

- Did you believe in things that other people don't believe in? Like what?
- Has there ever been a time your imagination played tricks on you? What kinds of tricks? Tell me more about them.
- Do you have any ideas about things that you don't tell anyone because you are afraid they might not understand? Like what?
- When you were with people you did not know, did you think that they are talking about you?
- Has there ever been a time you felt that someone was out to hurt you or make things difficult for you? Who? Why?
- Did you ever feel like you were being controlled by another person?
- Did you ever think you were an important or great person?
- Did you ever feel convinced that the world was coming to an end?
- Do you think that other people can hear your thoughts, or are putting thoughts into your head?

Chapter 7
Treatment

Previous chapters delineate the prevalence rates and trajectories for young people diagnosed with early-onset schizophrenia (EOS), theoretical orientations to understand its origins and development, as well as assessment strategies for screening, diagnosis, and psychoeducational purposes. EOS presents a complex challenge for mental health professionals in terms of its defining characteristics, and this complexity carries over to accompanying treatments. Because symptoms typically develop gradually, by the time affected children are referred for treatment, they may present severe characteristics of the disorder. Moreover, multiple inaccurate diagnoses may have been proffered before the correct identification occurs (Frazier et al., 2007; Schaeffer & Ross, 2002). As such, valuable time may have been lost in which an effective treatment approach could have been implemented. As discussed extensively in Chapter 3 and 5, the long-term prognosis of individuals affected by EOS is disconcerting. Nearly 70% of individuals continue to exhibit schizophrenia tendencies several years after treatment implementation began, with poorer outcomes associated with the length of time that psychosis exists in an individual prior to receiving treatment for schizophrenia (Asarnow, Tompson, & McGrath, 2004). Therefore, when developing a treatment plan for EOS, it is essential to expedite the delivery of services while also considering the child's developmental history, experience with mental health services, and desired developmental outcomes.

Treatment that remediates symptoms of schizophrenia brings with it the hope of a better outcome and the possibility of living a functional life. For the child with schizophrenia, there are serious long-term implications regarding his or her ability to function in every day life (e.g., self-care, employment, social relationships), especially as these symptoms continue into adulthood (Asarnow et al., 2004; Remschmidt & Theisen, 2005). Effective treatment may substantially decrease the long-term morbidity, decrease chronicity, and increase the potential for optimal response and outcome (Bryden, Carrey, & Kutcher, 2001). Effective treatment for EOS must be global and all-encompassing just as the symptoms of EOS fully encompass a young person's life (Sikich, 2005). This means targeting treatment for the specific phase of the disorder, and also providing treatment in a variety of settings with the involvement of various members of a child's team, including family members, educators, doctors, therapists, and other related professionals and

H. Li et al., *Identifying, Assessing, and Treating Early Onset Schizophrenia at School*,
Developmental Psychopathology at School, DOI 10.1007/978-1-4419-6272-0_7,

community supports. Treatment strategies must take the specific child into consideration and be individualized to promote treatment compliance and follow-through (Findling & Schulz, 2005).

In recent years, there have been considerable advancements in the treatment of schizophrenia. Contemporary treatments, including some form of pharmacotherapy with psychosocial interventions, may ameliorate the positive symptoms and improve quality of life (US Department of Health and Human Services-DHHS, 1999). The Schizophrenia Patient Outcomes Research Team (PORT), an expert panel sponsored by the Agency for Health Care and Research of the National Institutes of Mental Health (NIMH) and the DHHS, systematically reviewed the extant literature on scientifically proven treatments and identified 20 pharmacological and psychosocial state-of-the-art interventions (Lehman et al., 2004). These interventions focus primarily on the adult population with schizophrenia, as there are very few controlled trials that explicitly address treatment for children and adolescents with EOS. Given that child- and early-onset schizophrenia has been found to be continuous with adult-onset schizophrenia, treatments that are effective in adults may be effective in children as well, particularly when altered to address the developmental needs of children (American Academy of Child and Adolescent Psychiatry, 2001). As with adult treatments, adherence to treatment guidelines vary based on demographic and contextual variables (e.g., rural vs. urban, minority vs. whites), and "underscore the importance of identifying effective interventions, developing strategies for disseminating effective treatments into usual practice settings, and decreasing disparities in quality of care across diverse settings and patient groups" (Asarnow et al., 2004, p. 184).

Whether the treatment goals focus on the development of education, social, or daily living skills, school professionals can organize, provide, and facilitate a range of interventions that address symptoms and problematic behaviors that create the most difficulty for functioning in school and in daily life. This chapter articulates current evidence-based treatments, developmental considerations, as well as biological, behavioral, and educational treatment strategies that specifically relate to the unique role of school professionals.

Treatment Considerations

There are multiple factors that need to be considered when organizing school-based treatment strategies for a student with EOS. Treatment considerations include the ontogenic factors of the child, such as their developmental level, as well as dynamic factors of the illness. These factors are not stagnant, and therefore, will need to be revisited over the course of the student's educational planning.

Developmental Considerations

Due to the early and relatively severe nature of EOS, special consideration regarding the child's developmental level is warranted, as the challenges in distinguishing diagnoses carry over into matching appropriate treatment with the functional impairment. For instance, there are multiple developmental concerns related to the use of psychopharmacological agents with children, since medication efficacy and appropriateness may be seriously impacted by the influence of developmental pharmacodynamics on the response to antipsychotics (Bryden et al., 2001). This may include the effect of medications on a child's immature central nervous system as well as the interaction of hormonal changes (e.g., during puberty) with the pharmacological properties of medications. Additionally, traditional side effects of certain agents, such as weight gain and sedation, may impact treatment compliance and appropriateness of certain medications. Weight gain in particular may impact treatment adherence in adolescents as it relates to images of self-esteem and self-worth. Sedation can also seriously impact the developmental level of a child in relation to his/her ability to independently function in different learning and social environments such as school and the community. The use of psychopharmacological interventions requires frequent and consistent monitoring by health professionals to ensure healthy development for the child challenged by EOS.

The ability to fully understand and benefit from individualized treatment and psychosocial interventions will be impacted by a child's developmental stage. Psychosocial treatments must target the child's present level of functioning and build on them while also supporting the expansion of normative developmental experiences, such as social engagement and independent functioning. Treatments such as cognitive behavioral therapy and some aspects of psychoeducational treatment may not be appropriate for very young children who are not sufficiently cognitively aware to participate in these treatments (Asarnow et al., 2004). These types of treatments require some understanding of one's own thoughts, behaviors, and belief systems as they relate to the outside environment – an understanding even typically-developing children of a young age may not be able to grasp. If these treatment components are used, modifications may be needed to help children better understand them at their own cognitive and developmental level. Furthermore, unlike adult-onset schizophrenia, children with the disorder may not acquire many of the basic language, social, and daily living skills that are needed to function independently in everyday life. Rather than recapturing lost skills, children require timely and intensive interventions across settings (in the home, community, and school) that address the acquisition of new skills (Frazier et al., 2007).

Skills training targeted specifically at skills that have not been developed or acquired by children with schizophrenia should be chosen with the goal of facilitating better outcomes in the immediate as well as into later adulthood. Thus, in the school-based setting, the interventions can focus directly on issues related to the childhood-onset form of the disorder (e.g., academic and social functioning). Specialized educational services are needed to help children with EOS maintain a basic level of academic skills, as the ability to function independently in the school setting is lost very early in a child's academic career. Specialized, intensive support services, starting as early as the premorbid phase (see Chapter 5 for further discussion of the phases of EOS), are required throughout much of a child's school experience.

The very early nature of the disorder places primary importance on the role of the family in treatment. Here too, the developmental role of the child's place within the family structure may impact treatment appropriateness and efficacy. Any treatment component must fit into the family system and allow the child to function within that system. Family therapies are important in treating adults, yet this type of treatment is very important for young children whose parents tend to be the primary caregivers. Educational components address the possible progression of EOS, its impact on the child's development, and ways in which the family may cope with the developmental challenges.

Multi-Phase Considerations

Managing EOS symptoms is an ongoing and dynamic process. Asarnow et al. (2004), in their review of the treatment literature, outlined a practical three-phase model of treatment. This multi-phasic, multi-modal approach provides beneficial guidelines for mental health service providers, including school personnel, with respect to understanding the anticipated treatment process of youth affected by EOS. Again, a developmental perspective may be observed within this treatment approach in that the affected individual's developmental trajectory of symptom reduction and ultimate outcome is the primary focus. The three phases and treatment goals, as outlined by Asarnow et al. (2004, p. 184) and Kelsey, Newport and Nemeroff (2006) include:

1. During the **acute** phase, the emphasis is on bringing acute psychotic symptoms under control through a combination of medication and inpatient care, which is necessary during the first acute episode to rule out serious medical causes of psychosis,
2. During the **recovery (stabilization)** phase, outpatient pharmacologic and psychosocial treatment is employed with the goal of stabilizing the youth's clinical state, and
3. During the residual (**maintenance**) phase, the emphasis is on helping the youth to maintain a stable state through continuing multimodal treatment.

Treatments will vary based on the phase of illness; for example, cognitive-behavioral strategies that are helpful in the stabilization phase are not effective during periods of acute psychosis. During the acute phase, a child may display positive symptoms that indicate compromised judgment with the subsequent risk of harm to themselves or others – even though this harm may be an inadvertent consequence to their actively psychotic state (Kronenberger & Meyer, 2001). The focus on pharmacological interventions (discussed below) during the acute phase is not typically within the purview of school personnel; however, situations such as these may require school personnel to follow their system's crisis procedures to maintain the safety of all parties. During this critical window, school personnel can also facilitate the connection of the student with coordinated community and hospital providers to ensure effective treatment interventions. During the stabilization and maintenance phases, there is increased focus on the psychosocial interventions that can be carried out by community providers as well as school-based personnel. These interventions are discussed in more depth below.

Evidence-Based Treatments

As noted previously in this chapter, most of what is known about psychosocial and psychopharmacological treatments of schizophrenia is based on studies of adults. Brown et al. (2008) highlighted that (a) there are no clinical trials of psychosocial interventions including children with EOS, (b) there is one historical control study of adolescents with EOS suggesting that psychoeducationally oriented comprehensive care may be beneficial, (c) there are multiple studies examining the effects of psychopharmacological interventions (i.e., haloperidol, clozapine, risperidone, and olanzapine) for youth with psychotic symptoms, although not necessarily schizophrenia spectrum disorders, (d) that most psychopharmacological studies focus on acute symptoms, not long term outcomes, and (e) there are very few psychopharmacological studies of EOS including children under the age of 13 years. With these caveats, the following is a review of the literature pertaining to the treatment of adults and youth with schizophrenia.

Pharmacological Interventions

Advances in psychopharmacological treatment have been remarkable and the frontline of care is pharmacological treatment, as it has been shown to reduce positive symptoms and relapse rates in adults with schizophrenia (Ayuso-Gutierrez & del Rio, 1997; Lehman et al., 2004). The history of these medications begins with the serendipitous discovery of Thorazine in 1952, following by the introduction of about 15 new antipsychotic medications between 1954 and 1975, and the new era of atypical antipsychotic medications in 1990 (Shen, 1999). Though medical treatment is not the expertise of school personnel, school psychologists and school nurses can play a critical role in monitoring the effectiveness and side effects of pharmacological interventions, particularly when they are being introduced into the child's treatment and when these children are able to be in school. Collaboration between medical providers and school nurses and/or other school-based health personnel can assist with any dispersing of medications during this school day. School personnel are also in position to conduct observations in the naturalistic setting and communicate findings with medical providers, assuming that relevant parties have parental permission to communicate about the child's illness. Reporting observations is a critical role of the school psychologists, and from this perspective, a basic familiarity with these medications in the efficacious treatment of children and adolescents with schizophrenia is recommended.

For any pharmacological agent that is to be used in the treatment of children and adolescents, clear and strict guidelines should be followed. In its practice parameters for the treatment of EOS, the AACAP recommends that any medication tried with children be given a trial of at least 4–6 weeks to determine the efficacy of the medication. Only after this initial period of time should another antipsychotic agent be tried (AACAP, 2001). Dosage levels initially start small so that side effects may be minimized and monitoring schedules are ongoing and strictly required to detect any detrimental effects of the medications. Dosages, similar to other treatments, are modified based on whether the individual is in an acute or residual (maintenance) level of treatment (Lehman et al., 2004). Caregivers and health care providers carefully weigh the risks and benefits of the treatment outcomes and potential side effects. For some children and families, the risks may be minimal compared to the reduction of symptoms.

The use of pharmacological agents in the treatment of schizophrenia generally targets three areas: (a) control psychotic symptoms during the acute phase of the disorder (b) prevent relapse during the recovery and residual phases of the disorder, and (c) control side-effects (Remschmidt & Theisen, 2005). Given the severe side effects of many of the pharmacological agents (e.g., weight gain that may lead to Type 2 diabetes, problems with word retrieval, working memory, involuntary movements, prolactin elevation, intercardiac conduction effects, an neuroleptic malignant syndrome), their use is typically not recommended until the presentation of psychotic symptoms during the acute phase. Careful monitoring is suggested during the less severe prodromal phase of the disorder. Although the vast majority of current research on the use of antipsychotic agents to treat schizophrenia has been with adults, and some reports indicate that a higher percentage of children do not respond to medications, some research has shown that these agents may be effective in reducing symptoms in children (Armenteros & Davies, 2006; Bryden et al., 2001; Clark & Lewis, 1998). Roughly 70% of adult patients in the acute phase of illness experience a reduction of positive symptoms with conventional antipsychotic medications (Dixon, Lehman, & Levine, 1995).

There is no definitive consensus on whether first- or second-generation antipsychotic medications are more efficacious in the treatment of acute symptom; instead treatment is determined "on the basis of prior individual treatment response, relevant medical history, preferences, medication side effect profile, and long-term treatment planning" (Lehman et al., 2004, p. 196). The first generation antipsychotics, which are also referred to as conventional antipsychotics, classical neuroleptics, or major tranquilizers, include haloperidol, fluphenazine, and zuclopenthixol. This class of medications can lead to extrapyramidal side effects such as dystonia (involuntary movements and muscle contractions resulting in body motion, tremor, and abnormal posture), Parkinsonism, tardive dyskinesia (repetitive and involuntary movements such as grimacing, tongue protrusion, or rapid eye blinking), and neuroleptic malignment syndrome (NMS) (a life threatening neurological disorder—high fever, sweating, unstable blood pressure, and muscle rigidity). The second generation of antipsychotics, or atypical antipsychotics, (e.g., risperidone, aripiprazole, olanzapine, quetiapine) are equally effective and are associated with reduced extrapyramidal side effects, but have other side effects such as weight gain, neurological side effects, hypokinesia/akinesia (abnormally diminished motor activity), and dystonia (Castro-Fornieles et al., 2008). The last line of pharmacological treatment is clozapine, which is recommended for patients with treatment-resistant schizophrenia to reduce positive symptoms, hostility, and suicidality in addition to reducing other extrapyramidal symptoms such as tardive dyskinesia, NMS, or persistent dystonia (Lehman et al., 2004). Due to the risk of serious adverse effects associated with clozapine, a child would typically be treated with at least two conventional antipsychotics prior to this medication (Asarnow et al., 2004).

Limited systematic data exist on the use of these agents in children, though recent randomized, controlled trials on younger populations have been conducted that compare the use of antipsychotics with placebos, and comparing first- and second-generation antipsychotics. Findling et al. (2008) found a reduction in symptoms for children and adolescents with schizophrenia when comparing atypical antipsychotics to placebo. However, Sikich et al. (2008) concluded that the first- and second-generation antipsychotics are equally effective in younger populations, but that overall, the effectiveness is low. Recent concerns have focused on the increased use of second-generation antipsychotics with the side effect of weight gain combined with the greater risk for obesity in children, particularly since adults with schizophrenia have an increased prevalence of adult-onset Type-2 diabetes (Shin, Bregman, Frazier, & Noyes, 2008).

In a study by Armenteros, Whitaker, Welikerson, Stedge, and Gorman (1997), risperidone was shown to be effective in reducing symptoms of schizophrenia in 10 adolescents. Similarly, olanzapine was found to have an effect on both positive (agitation, delusions and hallucinations) and negative symptoms (anhedonia, affective bluntness, and social withdrawal) in nine chronic treatment-resistant children with early-onset schizophrenia (Mozes, Spivak, Tyano, Weizman, & Mester, 2003). In this same study, a reduction of at least 20% was noted in scores on all psychopathology scales as indicated by the *Brief Psychiatric Rating Scale* (BPRS), *Positive and Negative Syndrome Scale* (PANSS), and *Clinical Global Impression* (CGI). Common side-effects noted with these medications include weight gain and somnolence or sedation. Although not as severe as some of the side-effects noted with the traditional neuroleptics, these side-effects may also become an issue especially given the specific developmental phase of the child taking the medication. In particular, weight gain may become a concern for adolescents on the medication and may relate to medication compliance. The implications of sedation may be a cause for concern as well, given its influence on a child's ability to attend to tasks and the effect this may have on learning, school performance, work performance, and general social interaction (Bryden et al., 2001). Special consideration should be given to the potential influence these side effects may have on a child's ability to function at school, at home, and in the community.

Clozapine, also an atypical antipsychotic, has consistently been shown to be effective for adults with treatment refractory schizophrenia and has been shown by numerous studies to have an effect on the positive and negative symptoms of schizophrenia in children (Asarnow et al., 2004; Kranzler et al., 2005). In a study by Kranzler et al. (2005), clozapine use in adolescents in inpatient care was associated with a significant decrease in aggressive and violent episodes as measured by the number of incidents of seclusion and administration of emergency oral or injectable as needed medications. In general, clozapine appears to be very effective for children with treatment-resistant schizophrenia and those with chronic schizophrenia (Asarnow et al., 2004). Despite these advantages in the use of clozapine, this drug is generally not considered first-choice with children and adolescents due to the severe associated side effects. Side effects of this drug include seizures, neutropenia, granulocytopenia and agranulocytosis, and myocarditis. Data from a NIMH study on children with schizophrenia found that 38% (eight out of 21) of children given the drug clozapine developed neutropenia and/or seizures or were nonresponsive to treatment (AACAP, 2001). Given these side-effects, clozapine is typically used with children only after the failure to respond to two therapeutic trials of other antipsychotic agents (including at least one atypical antipsychotic agent) or when significant side effects have developed with other agents. Even then, weekly blood monitoring is recommended (AACAP, 2001). Table 7.1 provides a summary of antipsychotic medications, their generic and brand names as well as typical tablet dosage.

Despite the improved outcomes demonstrated on the positive symptoms of EOS, there currently are not similar outcomes for the treatment of the negative symptoms (e.g., asociality, anhedonia). Limited benefits from pharmacological treatments are evident, and according to Erhart, Marder, and Carpenter (2006), "a decade of accumulated data from intervention studies reveals inconsistencies in the pattern of responsiveness among negative symptoms" (p. 235). To date, the response to treatment of negative symptoms has "remained elusive" (p. 235).

In summary, a number of antipsychotic medications have been studied with adults over the past few decades with a more recent focus on their use and outcomes with younger populations. This section presented some basic information about antipsychotic medications and the extrapyramidal side effects that may be demonstrated. For further valuable information regarding various antipsychotic medications, the reader is referred to Lehman et al. (2004), Mozes et al. (2003), Ross, Novins, Farley, and Adler (2003), Findling et al. (2008), and Sikich et al. (2008).

Psychosocial Interventions

As previously mentioned, scientifically proven treatments and practice guidelines for adults with schizophrenia have been consolidated by the expert panel Schizophrenia Patient Outcomes Research Team (PORT; Lehman et al., 2004). The compilation of findings resulted in 20 treatment recommendations; 14 of which specifically target pharmacological interventions with the remaining six focusing on psychosocial interventions. Used in combination with pharmacological treatment, a number of psychosocial interventions have demonstrated positive effects on relapse rate, symptoms, and

Table 7.1 Antipsychotic Medications, Generic and Brand Names and Typical Tablet Dosage (Adapted from Wilens 2009)

	Generic Name	Brand Name	Tablet Dosage Range
Atypical	Risperidone	Risperdal	1–3 mg
	Olanzapine	Zyprexa	2.5–10 mg
	Clozapine	Clozaril	25–100 mg
	Quetiapine	Seroquel	25–200 mg
	Ziprasidone	Geodon	20–60 mg
	Aripiprazole	Abilify	5–15 mg
High potency typical	Haloperidol	Haldol	0.5–20 mg
	Pimozide	Orap	2 mg
	Fluphenazine	Prolixin	2.5–10 mg
Medium potency typical	Trifluoperazine	Stelazine	1–10 mg
	Perphenazine	Trilafon	2–16 mg
	Thiothixene	Navane	2–20 mg
	Loxapine	Loxitane	5–50 mg
Low potency typical	Molindone	Moban	5–100 mg
	Mesoridazine	Serentil	10–100 mg
	Thioridazine	Mellaril	10–200 mg
	Chlorpromazine	Thorazine	10–200 mg

social impairment among adults with schizophrenia (Drury, Birchwood, & Cochrane, 2000; Garety, Fowler, & Kuipers, 2000; Garety & Freeman, 1999; Hogarty & Ulrich, 1998; Lehman et al., 2004; Pinto, La Pia, Mennella, Giorgio, & DeSimone, 1999). Psychosocial interventions specifically target the stabilization and maintenance phases of the illness and complement pharmacological treatment. Despite the profound improvements noted for many individuals with schizophrenia, there are a number of limitations to pharmacological treatment alone, including: suboptimal compliance with medication regiment, which occurs in 45–60% with adult outpatient population (Fenton, Blyler, & Heinssen, 1997); positive symptoms that persist with 25–50% of those with schizophrenia (Wiersma, Nienhuis, & Stooff, 1998); and limited evidence that medications significantly improve social functioning, which is one of the strongest predictors of long-term outcomes (Amminger et al., 1999; Penn et al., 2004).

Similar to the pharmacological treatment of schizophrenia, much of the research relating to the efficacy of psychosocial treatments has centered on adults (Dulmus & Smyth, 2000; Haugaard, 2004). There is an urgent need for controlled studies evaluating the effectiveness of psychosocial treatments with children and adolescents as there are "no published randomized controlled trials evaluating psychosocial treatments for schizophrenia in youth" (Asarnow et al., 2004, p. 184). The psychosocial treatments reviewed in this section present developmental modification of the recommendations from the PORT expert panel (Lehman et al., 2004) as well as build on the review of childhood focused treatments by Asarnow et al. (2004). These treatments focus on the needs of children and adolescents with schizophrenia as it impacts their functioning in school and community-based settings. As such, the strategies target the individual, the family, and the systems that support them as they manage this illness. These strategies are outlined in Table 7.2.

Table 7.2 Targets And Key Elements of Recommended Psychosocial Interventions

Target	Recommendation	Key Elements
Cognitive Behaviorally oriented Psychotherapy	Persons with schizophrenia who have residual psychotic symptoms while receiving adequate pharmacotherapy should be offered adjunctive cognitive behaviorally oriented psychotherapy	• Shared understanding of the illness between the patient and therapist • Identification of target symptoms • Development of specific cognitive and behavioral strategies to cope with these symptoms
Skills training	Persons with schizophrenia who have skill deficits such as problems with social skills or activities of daily living should be offered skills training	• Behaviorally based instruction • Modeling • Corrective feedback • Contingent social reinforcement • Clinic-based skills training should be supplemented with practice and training in the individual's day-to-day environment
Family intervention	Persons with schizophrenia and their families should be offered a family intervention	• Duration of at least 9 months • Crisis intervention • Emotional support • Training in how to cope with illness symptoms and related problems
Assertive community treatment (similar to the Wraparound model for youth)	Systems of care serving persons with schizophrenia should include a program of assertive community treatment (ACT). This intervention should be provided to individuals who have any of the following characteristics: high risk for repeated hospitalizations, difficulty remaining in traditional services, or recent homelessness	• Multidisciplinary team (including a psychiatrist and school personnel) • Shared caseload among team members • Direct service provision by team members • High frequency of patient contact • Low patient-to-staff ratios • Outreach to patients in the community
Supported employment and education	Persons with schizophrenia who have the goal of employment should be offered supported employment and education	• Individualized job development and educational goals • Rapid placement emphasizing competitive employment • Ongoing job and academic support • Integration of vocational, educational, and mental health services
Tokeneconomy interventions in classroom-based behavioral programming	Systems of care that deliver long-term inpatient or residential care should provide a behavioral intervention based on social learning principles, often referred to as a token economy	• Contingent positive reinforcement for clearly defined target behaviors • Individualized treatment approach • Avoidance of punishing consequences

Cognitive-Behavioral Therapy

Cognitive Behavioral Therapy (CBT) focuses on the thoughts, emotions, and behaviors associated with symptoms of the disorder, as well as triggers, consequences, and responses to symptoms. Cognitive behavioral interventions focus on identification of target symptoms, strategies to cope with these symptoms, interpretations of reality, affect regulation, and recognition of sources and signs of stress (Asarnow et al., 2004; Lehman et al., 2004; Penn et al., 2004). The benefits of CBT are most profound for those who have persistent symptoms despite ongoing and adequate medication treatment, though it does not bestow the same advantage to those who are in the acute phase of illness (Dickerson, 2000).

CBT interventions involve active collaboration between the child and treatment provider. The treatment begins "with a thorough evaluation of the psychotic symptoms and the emotions, thoughts and behaviors which accompany the symptoms, the triggers/context for the occurrence of symptoms, their consequences, and nature and effectiveness of attempts to cope with them" (Asarnow et al., 2004, p. 187). In creating a shared understanding of the illness, psychoeducational treatment for the child includes specific education about the nature of the disorder, the importance of treatment compliance, treatment options, and relapse prevention (Dilk & Bond, 1996). This type of intervention may be best suited for older children and adolescents with higher cognitive functioning and capacities or it requires that the treatment be considerably modified; as an example, with an 11-year-old, strategies can be adapted to match the cognitive and language levels of the child by using simple instructions and self-talk scripts that are concrete and short (Sikich, 2005). Strategies with children include modeling techniques, such as role playing, reinforcing, and mirroring – and can include strategies such as watching videotapes of a similarly-aged child who is competent but not highly skilled at the task being taught (Bandura, 1977; Sikich, 2005). Similar to adult CBT, goals and objectives of treatment must be tailored to meet the needs and preferences of each individual – though areas of growth can be identified by the caretakers rather than the child.

Evidence-based treatments that complement the psychoeducational components of CBT are Supportive Therapy, as discussed by Penn et al. (2004), and Personal Therapy, as described by Hogarty (2002). The strategies of Supportive Therapy focus on the therapeutic alliance, the provision of support and advice, and the efforts to minimize stress. Similarly, Personal Therapy emphasizes support, education, and skill building to increase personal competence at self-regulation and to develop self-awareness regarding affective, cognitive, and behavioral states.

Like adults, children or adolescents with schizophrenia may be especially responsive to the nonspecific elements of a supportive therapeutic relationship, yet this may be especially applicable if the professional providing this support is accessible to them in their daily life, such as within the school community. With the impoverished social networks and need for social contact associated with these symptoms, supportive strategies can help bring the youth back into the social world (Davidson, Stayner, & Haglund, 1998). This support can mitigate stressful circumstances that the individual encounters during the social and academic challenges of school, again highlighting the unique role that school professionals can play in supporting a young person with EOS.

Skills Training

The premorbid abnormalities and early onset of psychotic symptoms found in children and adolescents with EOS often lead to a severe disruption in the child's global development (see Chapter 3 for further discussion of premorbid and comorbid considerations). Skill deficits in numerous domains often exist due to the child's inability to develop or acquire new skills during the early stages of the disorder. Given the difficulties associated with these deficits in functioning, a major component in the treatment of schizophrenia in children should focus on the practical, everyday aspects of the disorder. Skills training that focuses on communication skills, social skills, and daily life skills are essential components in early treatment of children with EOS (AACAP, 2001; Asarnow et al., 2004; Gonthier & Lyon, 2004). Skills training groups that have been found to be most effective have included behaviorally-based instruction that includes components such as modeling, corrective feedback, and the use of contingent social reinforcements and reward systems (Dulmus & Smyth, 2000).

Skills training in adults has been shown to be effective in remediating some associated symptoms of the disorder and better social adjustment (see review in Dulmus & Smyth, 2000). For children and adolescents, skills training should focus on learning age-appropriate skills needed to function in their social environment such as learning conversational skills, basic self-care skills, and money management skills. Sikich (2005) also recommends that social skills training should focus on nonverbal behavior, such as eye contact, posture, facial expression, tone, and volume of speech, all which impact functioning in social situations. The acquisition of new skills may occur in a small group setting with targeted strategies to support generalization to other settings, again highlighting the unique opportunities for the school setting to provide the opportunity for generalization to multiple environments, such as classroom, lunch room, and transition times. Additionally, family members should be provided with basic information about the illness given their caretaking role for children and adolescents.

Research has demonstrated that social skills training improves functioning in the targeted areas, yet despite this success, there are concerns about the generalization of these skills and what, if any, impact they have on general functioning (Benton & Schroeder, 1990; Mueser & Bond, 2000). Furthermore, social skills training has demonstrated little impact on the risk of relapse, symptom severity, global adjustment, or quality of life, thus making little to no impact on the negative symptoms (Pilling et al., 2002). Outcomes are most promising when there is a combination of psychopharmacological interventions with CBT and skills training. In a study combining these treatments for those with treatment refractory schizophrenia (Pinto et al., 1999), there were significant improvements in positive symptoms and none of the participants experiences relapse.

Family Interventions

A particularly salient aspect of EOS is its influence on the family. Family involvement is an important treatment strategy when treating adults with schizophrenia, as a meta-analytic study by Pilling et al. (2002) demonstrated that family therapy significantly prevented psychotic relapses and readmissions to psychiatric hospitals, reduced family burden, and improved treatment adherence. These findings indicate that families can have a significant positive impact on individuals affected by schizophrenia. Yet, family involvement and intervention become particularly critical when treating a child with EOS as they most likely reside with their family and are dependent upon them to support and access treatment (Asarnow et al., 2004). Family-focused interventions require an understanding of this system, particularly since familial studies have indicated that parents of individuals with EOS have higher rates of schizophrenia and schizophrenia spectrum disorders than parents of patients with adult-onset illness, and relatives of children and adolescents with ADHD (Margari et al., 2008; Nicolson et al., 2003). Parents of youth with EOS also experience higher levels of social isolation, introversion, suspiciousness, and hostility than parents of children with autism and ADHD (Nicolson et al., 2003).

Environmental stressors have been shown to be a factor in adult patient relapse and a strong positive association has been found between level of expressed emotion (e.g., overly critical, hostile, overinvolved and highly emotionally expressive family style) within the family and child outcome and relapse (Dulmus & Smyth, 2000; Gonthier & Lyon, 2004). When families participate in the treatment, many positive outcomes have been demonstrated, such as improved family problem-solving and enhanced psychosocial functioning (Doane, Goldstein, Miklowitz, & Falloon, 1986; Hogarty, 2002). Given these findings in adult and child populations, it appears that any treatment package that is to be effective in reducing child symptomatology must include a family treatment component. The critical components of effective family intervention programs have been organized by Goldstein and Miklowitz (1995) and are listed in Table 7.3.

Family therapy should be targeted at reducing the environmental stressors brought on by the disorder so as to reduce the likelihood of relapse (Clark & Lewis, 1998). This can include educating the family members about the illness as well as behavior management strategies (e.g., lecture, role playing, modeling, rehearsal, and homework) aimed at understanding the nature of the disorder, developing coping strategies, and strengthening problem solving skills and basic communication skills. Training and support around how to handle crisis situations, such as when the child's reality testing becomes so compromised that they are at risk of hurting themselves or others, is also an important part of family treatment (Tomoras et al., 2000).

Psychoeducationally focused family treatment can be organized as a single-family unit or as part of multiple-family groups. Yet, noteworthy findings by McFarlane et al. (1995) demonstrated that multiple-family groups had significantly lower relapse rates than single-family groups. Whether the family engages in the treatment as a single unit, or as part of a group, programs lasting at least 9 months

Table 7.3 Common Ingredients in Effective Family Intervention Programs (Reprinted from Goldstein & Miklowitz, 1995. With permission)

1. Engagement of the family early in the treatment process in a no-fault atmosphere
2. Education about schizophrenia concerning:
   - The vulnerability-stress model
   - Etiologic theories
   - Variations in prognosis
   - Rationale for various treatments
3. Recommendations for coping with the disorder
4. Communication training directed at improving:
   - Communication clarity in general
   - Ways of providing positive and negative feedback within the family
5. Problem-solving training directed at improving:
   - Management of day-to-day problems and hassles
   - Management of discrete stressful life events
   - Generalized problem-solving skills
6. Crisis intervention:
   - In times of extreme stress involving one or more members of the family
   - When incipient signs of recurrence are evident

demonstrate more positive outcomes, and those lasting less than 6 months have little effect (Pitschel-Walz, Leucht, Bauml, Kissling, & Engel, 2001), again substantiating the chronicity and long-term adjustment associated with this disorder.

Assertive Community Treatment and Wrap-Around Services

Addressing the needs of a child or adolescent with EOS requires interventions at multisystemic levels. Randomized trials support the efficacy of *Assertive Community Treatment* (ACT; Burns & Santos, 1995) described as "a way of delivering comprehensive and effective services to individuals who are diagnosed with severe mental illness and who have needs that have not been well met by traditional approaches to delivering services" (U.S. DHHS, n.d.).This community-based treatment is provided by transdisciplinary teams that collaborate on assessments, treatment planning, and day-to-day interventions. Comprehensive services are individualized and carried out in the community with treatment and support available 24 hour a day.

The *ACT* service delivery model has been recommended by the Schizophrenia PORT (Lehman et al., 2004); however, this model is adult focused – as evidenced by its application to areas such as independent living and employment. The same System of Care movement has been instrumental in the development of community-based services and supports for *children and adolescents* with serious and profound mental illness, such as schizophrenia. In 1992, the *Comprehensive Community Mental Health Services for Children and Their Families Program* (P.L. 102-321) was created, based on the Systems of Care model, and dedicated to coordinating service providers from multiple systems to develop a cohesive plan to support children with mental health impairments to stay in the home and community

(Kendziora, Bruns, Osher, Pacchiano, & Mejia, 2001). In contrast to the typical clinical model (e.g., weekly office appointments, fragmented services), this model relies on the family and assists in identifying "natural supports," subsequently improving functioning in the community and relying less on professionals (Worthington, Hernandez, Friedman, & Uzzell, 2001).

These services, typically referred to as Wraparound and similar to *ACT*, involve the child and family in the planning process, maintain a strengths-based focus, utilize community-based resources and supports, and tend to be operated by community mental health centers (Walker, 2008) with evidence to support its efficacy when implemented with fidelity (Bruns, 2008). Wraparound is a dynamic process based on an individualized, strength based and needs-driven service delivery model that is designed to support interagency collaboration as the team provides culturally competent services (US DHHS, 1999). Interagency cooperation is an integral part of this model with agencies providing services in the areas of mental health, education, social services, juvenile justice, and recreation.

Wraparound services are primarily initiated through mental health or child welfare systems, nonetheless they can result in improved outcomes in school performance (Eber, Sugai, Smith, & Scott, 2002). In a five site study of youth participating in Wraparound services (Taub & Pearrow, 2007), significant improvements were noted in several areas of school functioning, such as grades and access to support services. While this model supports interagency collaboration, the results of this study indicated that only half of these teams included school personnel. The best predictors of school personnel involvement included: age of child, level of impairment, and identification as needing special education services. The lack of school representation on these teams was concerning given the amount of time that these youth spent in school and the range and level of impairment required to qualify for the Wraparound services, thus suggesting the need for more representation from school personnel in the service delivery of children with serious mental illness.

Ideally, the services supporting the child or adolescent with schizophrenia occur in the community. However, given the severity of the disorder, placement of the child outside of the family home, especially during the acute phase of the disorder, may be a necessary condition of treatment. This may include day treatment programs or inpatient, residential facilities that provide a range of services tailored to meet the multidimensional and complex needs of the child with schizophrenia (Remschmidt, 2002). Additionally, close monitoring and supervision is available to ensure evaluation of treatment efficacy and adherence (Gonthier & Lyon, 2004). Children and adolescents are provided with a consistent and reliable routine that may reduce stress that may not be available in the natural, home environment. As with all treatment options, however, the effect on the child's well being must be closely monitored to ensure treatment efficacy. In particular, given a child's developmental stage and functioning, separation from family and home may not be the optimal strategy and may even result in negative outcomes. In all cases, the least restrictive setting ensuring optimal treatment effectiveness should be considered, whether that be in the home, in a day treatment setting or residential facility.

Psychoeducational Interventions in the School Setting

The four previous psychosocial interventions have strong empirical evidence but primarily involve treatment coordinated with mental health and community service agencies. The remaining three psychosocial interventions have strong applicability to the school setting. The first two have been identified by the Schizophrenia PORT (Lehman et al., 2004) as evidence-based practices, and the final one is supported by the NIMH and has been evaluated by Watson et al. (2004).

Supported employment and education. The Supported Employment treatment recommendation of the Schizophrenia PORT focuses on strategies such as individualized job development, ongoing job support, and integration of vocational and mental health services (Lehman et al., 2004). However, the "job" of children and adolescents is school; thus, the application of this intervention to the lives of youth requires modifications to address issues of educational and social development within the school environment. One noteworthy exception – Lehman et al. (2004) recommend that "any person with schizophrenia who expresses an interest in work should be offered supported employment" (p. 202). This applies to high school students with EOS. For children and adolescents, school is mandated and not a matter of choice. Strained social situations and missed school days can result in a young person with schizophrenia not wanting to participate in school; however, school professionals are in unique positions to make the environment and educational opportunities as welcoming as possible.

The special education federal regulation's definition of "emotional disturbance" specifically includes schizophrenia (see Chapter 1 and 6 for further discussion). This assumes that individuals affected with this low incidence disability will require additional support services that target academic as well as social, emotional, and behavioral supports available through special education programming. Eligibility for special education should consider functional ability in various phases of illness. In one recent case, one author worked with a 15-year-old boy who demonstrated high average to superior skills on achievement tests and was very successful academically when he was stable. However, during acute phases, he clearly demonstrated the need for organizational, social, and ancillary support services.

The goals of these support services may vary based on many factors, including the child's unique needs and the phase of the illness. Modifications in course content may be needed; for example, Sikich (2005) suggests that it is inappropriate for a psychotic child to read Kafka's *Metamorphosis*. An Individualized Education Program (IEP) for a student with schizophrenia may also include accommodations on attendance offering flexibility for doctors' appointments, hospitalizations, and recovery periods. Other supports may need to address organizational skills, daily living skills, and social skills – as discussed above. Some general examples of school-based modifications are listed in Table 7.4. These examples are generated based on anecdotal, clinical experience as well as reviewing multiple IEPs for students who experience significant and on-going struggles with reality testing. The empirical support to validate these as educational strategies is based on single case

Table 7.4 Examples of Modifications and Accommodations

Area of Vulnerability	Strategies and Supports
Daily activities	Homeroom assignment that provides specialized organizational and social support daily, including check-ins on hygiene and reality orientation Reminders of daily academic and social expectations Allowed to use gum or water as dryness of mouth can be a side-effect of medications Established firm limits on inappropriate behaviors
Reality testing	Access to support services during periods of stress Supportive feedback about perceptions Encouragement to focus on reality of external world Modified or altered academic assignments Gently confront illogical thoughts and speech
Academics	Study skills period to assist with organization Agenda books with daily calendar Academic assignments posted on school web site Repetition and clarification of material and assignments Use of visual and graphic organizers Shortened assignments, or assistance breaking down long-term assignments into smaller segments Tutoring Opportunity to repeat same class session if offered a second time (secondary school) Taking examinations in separate, quiet room
Attendance	Designed with flexibility to meet medical needs Option to complete assignments when out of school Permanent pass out of classes where there is a substitute teacher
Transition times	Partner with a peer Allowed to leave class early to transition with fewer people in hallways
Unstructured times	Participation in smaller setting for lunch Limiting participation in group assemblies
Peer relationships	Social skills training Peer support groups

designs, and implementation of these strategies should be accompanied by additional efforts to monitor the impact on academic and social development.

Declines in scholastic and academic achievement are noted in children and adolescents even during the early phases of the disorder (Asarnow et al., 2004). During the premorbid phase of the disorder, characterized by delays in language, social, and motor development, specific services may be required to assist children in school. These include, but are not limited to speech and language services, physical or occupational therapy, and the implementation of behavioral plans. As the disorder progresses and functioning begins to deteriorate, additional services, such as skills training programs may need to be implemented as well. As the more severe, psychotic symptoms begin to develop, additional, more focused services are likely to be required. Special accommodations such as smaller classroom settings and experienced teachers may be helpful in meeting the needs of a particular child's functioning level (AACAP, 2001). Additionally, other accommodations aimed at reducing stress, and decreasing frustration may include adjustments to the curriculum such as shorter assignments, breaking tasks into smaller pieces, tutoring, direct instruction, and designing assignments to ensure success (Gonthier & Lyon, 2004).

Additionally, school psychologists and school-based mental health professionals can assist in the integration of educational and mental health services. These professionals, trained in issues of confidentiality, can work as liaisons between community-based mental health providers and education personnel. They can provide guidance and assistance to teachers and administrators as they make programmatic and placement decisions to meet the needs of individuals with schizophrenia.

Token economy interventions in classroom-based behavioral programming. Within the context of controlled environments, a token economy system has demonstrated efficacy as it establishes clear expectations and consequences for behaviors (Lehman et al., 2004). Token economy systems, based on social learning theory, are comprehensive behavioral programs that provide positive reinforcement, in the form of tokens or points, for displaying targeted behaviors. They have proven to be flexible and effective interventions for children or adolescents with various disabilities, and this behavioral programming can be applied to the school setting to target academic and social skill development (Matson & Boisjoli, 2009). These tokens or points can also be taken away when inappropriate behaviors are demonstrated. They can be exchanged for particular rewards, based on the individual's preferences, or in the case of a classroom setting, can be exchanged for a group contingency reward (e.g., pizza party). In many ways, these interventions replicate the monetary economy in the community (Coleman, 1973). However, these interventions can be difficult to deliver and complex, as the school must ensure that there is "consistency among staff in carrying out a token economy program and in administering reinforcements to patients that are positive, immediate, and specific" (Dickerson, Tenhula, & Green-Paden, 2005, p. 414).

Token economy systems have demonstrated improvements on behavior, such as interpersonal skills, cooperation, and self-care, and reduced inappropriate behaviors such as rocking; however, they do not decrease bizarre cognitions or emotional behaviors, such as crying or screaming (Paul & Lentz, 1977). The effectiveness of token economy interventions is dependent upon issues such as staff training, client resistance, circumvention of the contingencies, and nonresponsiveness of subjects (Kazdin & Bootzin, 1972). Token economies are determined to be efficacious with adults with schizophrenia but more research is needed to determine the specific benefits of token economy systems with children with EOS, primarily since much of the research in this area is with adults in long-term care and performed more than 20 years ago and prior to the explosion of pharmacological interventions (Dickerson et al., 2005).

School-wide interventions. The impact of stigma and discrimination can have profound implications for youth in development as they struggle with mental illness on top of the typical identity issues (US DHHS, 1999). Schools are in a unique position to address issues of stigma and discrimination by educating youth with the facts of mental illness in general, schizophrenia in particular, as well as the requirements of treatment. To address this need, the National Institutes of Health (NIH) Office of Science Education and the NIMH sponsored the development of *The Science of Mental Illness* curriculum which targets middle school children. It introduces the concept that mental illnesses have a biological basis and are therefore not that different from other illnesses or diseases. The modules cover the development and identification of mental illness and targets specifically ADHD, depression, and schizophrenia. The module on schizophrenia addresses symptoms and causes in addition to information on accessing treatment. More information is available in the Appendix.

An evaluation of this program was conducted by Watson et al. (2004) after it was implemented with over 1,500 students in the United States indicating significant improvement in knowledge and attitudes regarding mental illness. A noteworthy outcome was that the curriculum was most effective in improving attitudes for those who initially indicated more negative attitudes. This suggests that, given the unique access that schools have to the general population, implementation of this curriculum can help reduce stigma and discrimination of mental illness.

Summary and Conclusions

School professionals, particularly those working as school psychologists and school counselors, can play an important role in directing families toward effective interventions. Given the range of misperceptions of causes and treatments, it is important that these professionals maintain accurate and scientifically-based information to support families as they navigate the complex medical, mental health, and education systems.

The optimal treatment for childhood-onset schizophrenia is multimodal. Each of the previously reviewed treatment approaches has benefits for a young person with EOS, and it is important to incorporate the various strategies to address the different symptoms and functional impairments faced by the child and family. The first line of treatment is usually pharmacological because of the debilitating effects of psychotic symptoms. Although there is research to show that neuroleptics and antipsychotics are less effective with children than with adults, there is also evidence to show that these drugs are effective in reducing psychotic symptoms for some children with EOS. To date, however, recovery from negative symptoms remains elusive (Erhart et al., 2006).

As discussed in this chapter, cognitive-behavioral therapy is the method of psychotherapy that has been shown to be the most effective in treating adults with schizophrenia. This type of intervention involves a close working relationship between the patient and therapist and active participation of the youth. Unfortunately, this therapy is restricted to older children and adolescents with higher cognitive functioning and capacities because of the cognitive capabilities required to benefit from the therapy.

A younger child would most likely not be able to understand and focus on the thoughts, emotions, and behaviors associated with symptoms of the disorder, nor the triggers, consequences, and responses to symptoms. Therefore, when the child with EOS is cognitively advanced enough, CBT is highly recommended to help him or her devise strategies to best cope with their symptoms, improve his or her capacity to test reality, monitor behavior, and alter dysfunctional beliefs and attributions.

Because EOS leads to a disruption of global functioning, psychoeducational treatment with skills training focusing on communication skills, social skills, and daily life skills are essential components of treatment (AACAP, 2001; Asarnow et al., 2004; Gonthier & Lyon, 2004; Lehman et al., 2004). Skills training should be sensitive to the developmental level of the child and targeted to the identified areas of impairment for the child with EOS, such as learning age appropriate conversational skills, basic self-care skills, and money management skills.

Incorporating the family into the treatment process is very beneficial for the youth with EOS because the family learns how to better interact with the child or adolescent, anticipate and deal with psychotic and negative symptoms, and provide emotional and psychological support for the child. Therefore, a multimodal treatment package must include a family treatment component if it is to be effective in reducing symptomatology. Family therapy should be targeted at reducing the environmental stressors brought on by the disorder so as to reduce the likelihood of relapse (Clark & Lewis, 1998). Strategies involved in family therapy may include family behavioral management strategies (including lecture, role playing, modeling, rehearsal, and homework) aimed at understanding the nature of the disorder, developing coping strategies, strengthening problem solving skills, and basic communication skills.

Systemic interventions, through interagency collaboration such as Wraparound, with coordinated services can implement cohesive plans to support youth with schizophrenia to stay in the home and community (Kendziora et al., 2001). However, depending upon the severity of the disorder, placement of the child outside of the family home, especially during the acute phase of the disorder, may be necessary. In all cases, the least restrictive setting ensuring optimal treatment effectiveness should be considered.

Interventions that target academic and social development in the school setting can help mitigate stress during various phases of the illness. School personnel can provide a range of supported educational practices and academic accommodations and provide optimal treatment by using token economy systems. Not only can schools support the individual with EOS in this setting, they also have the opportunity to educate the peer group to reduce stigma and discrimination.

Appendix

Early Onset Schizophrenia Resources

Valuable Information on the Internet

The Internet can be an important tool for parents, teachers, and professionals seeking information on Early Onset Schizophrenia and related topics. However, the preponderance of information that can be retrieved in any given search can also make it a time-consuming and unwieldy resource. To make the search more manageable, some useful websites are listed below. The following list is by no means exhaustive, but it contains links to some of the most valuable web-based materials that are currently available.

Epidemiology and General Information

National Institute of Mental Health

http://www.nimh.nih.gov/health/topics/schizophrenia/index.shtml

This site is the gateway to research-related information provided by the National Institute of Mental Health (NIMH). This site provides general information to the public about schizophrenia through easy to read publications and fact sheets; specific information is also provided about childhood-onset schizophrenia. Additionally, NIMH as an agency, continues to sponsor numerous studies related to a better understanding of the disorder, including a longitudinal study specific to COS initiated in 1990. There are numerous resources for a wide array of persons (e.g., individuals with schizophrenia, family members, scientists, professionals) providing the current research on the topic of COS related to various aspects of the disorder including etiology, assessment, and treatment.

MedlinePlus: Schizophrenia

http://www.nlm.nih.gov/medlineplus/schizophrenia.html

This site is one section of the larger website, MedlinePlus, sponsored by the U.S. National Library of Medicine (NLM) and the National Institutes of Health (NIH). This site offers valuable information for mental health professionals as well as the general public and shares information from governmental agencies, national organizations, and world organizations [including the National Library of Medicine (NLM), the National Institutes of Health (NIH), the American Psychiatric Association, and the World Fellowship for Schizophrenia and Allied Disorders]. Access to medical journal articles is provided and linked through the research database MEDLINE. Additionally, this site offers fact-sheets, information about drugs, an illustrated medical encyclopedia, and patient tutorials. The site provides information about diagnosis, symptoms, coping strategies, current research, clinical trials, and more through links to sites from reputable national agencies. Included among these links is information related specifically to schizophrenia in children. This website offers access to the most up-to-date information and research on the topic of schizophrenia. The focus of this site is on the dissemination of scientifically- and empirically-based research and evidence.

Mental Health Research Association

http://www.narsad.org/

This is the official site for the Mental Health Research Association (previously known as the National Alliance for Research on Schizophrenia and Depression). This is a nonprofit organization dedicated to supporting research on the causes, treatment, and prevention of psychiatric brain-based disorders. This site provides updated information and news about the various disorders, including schizophrenia, and highlights the most current research on the topic. This site may be useful to those interested in getting quick access to current research topics in schizophrenia as well as developing a better understanding of the particular disorder.

Schizophrenia.com: Information, Support, and Education

http://www.schizophrenia.com/index.php

Schizophrenia.com is a comprehensive site started in 1995 by family members of individuals diagnosed with schizophrenia. This site is described as a nonprofit web-community dedicated to the education and support of those impacted by schizophrenia. Schizophrenia.com includes schizophrenia-related information on a range of topics and the provision of support for individuals with the disorder, family members, and interested others. Although this site is not specific to early onset schizophrenia, information is provided related to this specific subgroup of individuals. Links and information on this site includes basic information about the disorder (e.g., definition, risk factors, prognosis, treatment) as well as news blogs, discussion groups, chat rooms, links to articles (based in newspapers and scientific journals), a newsletter, and even links to international discussion groups. Although the site is not affiliated with any particular mental health group, the site regularly consults with professionals and experts in the field, offering a list of consultants that have contributed. Schizophrenia.com provides information in a manner that may be easily accessed by the general public.

Assessment

National Institute of Mental Health Diagnostic Interview Schedule for Children (NIMH-DISC)

http://chipts.ucla.edu/assessment/pdf/assessments/disc_for_the_web.pdf

This document, which downloads as a PDF file, provides a brief description of the current versions of the National Institute of Mental Health Diagnostic Interview Schedule for Children ("NIMH-DISC" or "DISC"). The NIMH-DISC may be used for assessment. The NIMH DISC IV or "DISC" is a highly structured diagnostic interview used to assess psychiatric diagnoses of children and adolescents. The interview covers DSM-IV, DSMIII-R, and ICD-10, including over thirty common mental health disorders of children and adolescents. The DISC was designed to be administered by interviewers with no formal clinical training following the rules and conventions outlined in the DISC training manual.

Kiddie-Schedule for Affective Disorders and Schizophrenia-Present and Lifetime version (K-SADS-PL)

www.wpic.pitt.edu/ksads

This site is administered by the University of Pittsburgh's School of Medicine, Department of Psychiatry and provides direct access to the 2009 K-SADS-PL in PDF format. The K-SADS-PL is a semi-structured diagnostic interview designed to assess the presence of psychopathology in children and adolescents. Schizophrenia is one of the many disorders that may be diagnosed using this interview. Use of the instrument is permitted for clinical use in a nonprofit setting and in an IRB approved research protocol. The site also provides information about the administration of the K-SADS-PL for professionals.

Achenbach System of Empirically Based Assessment

www.aseba.org

Aseba.org is the home of the Achenbach System of Empirically Based Assessment as developed primarily by researchers at the Research Center for Children, Youth, and Families, Inc., directed by Thomas M. Achenbach, Ph.D. This center and site provide professionals with the tools to assess the adaptive and maladaptive functioning of children and adolescents through a variety of research-based assessments and instruments including the Child Behavior Checklist (CBCL). Although not specific to schizophrenia, scales within the instruments provide professionals with useful information regarding social, emotional, and behavioral functioning of youth. This site offers professionals access to information about ASEBA products and tools, ordering information, support resources as well as access to research updates related to ASEBA products.

Behavior Assessment System for Children, Second Edition: BASC-2

http://www.pearsonassessments.com/basc.aspx

This website provides an overview of the Behavior Assessment System for Children, Second Edition (BASC-2). While not specific to schizophrenia, the BASC-2 may help to understand the behaviors and emotions of children and adolescents. The BASC-2 includes a comprehensive set of rating scales and forms including the Teacher Rating Scales (TRS), Parent Rating Scales (PRS), Self-Report of Personality (SRP), Student Observation System (SOS), and Structured Developmental History (SDH). In addition to information about the development and use of the BASC-2, there is also a link to relevant publications.

The Positive and Negative Syndrome Scale (PANSS) Institute

http://www.panss.org/index.htm

This is the official site for The PANSS Institute (TPI) founded by the developers of the Positive and Negative Symptom Scale (PANSS). The PANSS is an instrument used to measure the symptoms of schizophrenia. This site shares information pertaining to training and certification in the use of the PANSS. This site also offers information about the scales and their use as well as information related to the development of this instrument. Although the site does not specifically address the Kiddie-PANSS, contact and support information provided through the site may help professionals access this diagnostic tool.

Rating Scales for Schizophrenia: Neurotransmitter.net

http://www.neurotransmitter.net/schizophreniascales.html

This website was established to provide biomedical information in fields such as neuroscience, pharmacology, and psychology. The site presents a wide variety of rating scales that may be utilized in the assessment of schizophrenia, including COS. Many of the rating scales are available via hyperlinks, thus, may be explored in greater detail to determine whether they would be appropriate. This site is geared toward mental health professionals who have been trained to administer these types of assessments and therefore, is not recommended to parents or others.

Children's Global Assessment Scale

http://depts.washington.edu/washinst/Resources/CGAS/CGAS%20Index.htm

This website describes the Children's Global Assessment Scale. A link to the Washington Institute On-Line Training and Assessment is also included. The site indicates that if used periodically, global assessment scales may serve as useful tools for planning treatment and measuring and predicting outcomes. The Children's Global Assessment Scale is a 100-point rating scale measuring psychological, social, and school functioning for children aged 6–17. It was adapted from the Adult Global Assessment Scale and is a tool for rating a child's general level of functioning on a health-illness continuum.

Advocacy and Family Support Resources

North American Society for Childhood Onset Schizophrenia

http://www.nascos.org/Home/

This site was developed by the North American Society for Childhood Onset Schizophrenia for the purpose of helping families and professionals share information and resources. Basic information specific to COS is provided for the general public. Family members and interested others are invited to become members of the site, which in turn allows access to the site's Knowledge Base. The Knowledge Base contains updated information on research and resources for parents and family members. Links to other schizophrenia-related sites are also provided.

Mental Health America

http://www.nmha.org/

The Mental Health America (formerly known as the National Mental Health Association, NMHA) site provides information about an array of mental disorders including schizophrenia. The NMHA aims to educate the general public about mental disorders and to support reform movements related to mental disorders. This site provides information describing various disorders, news about current research on various disorders, information related to advocacy, information about local chapters of NMHA, and information about local and national events centered on mental disorders. This site provides easy access to information but is limited in information specific to EOS.

World Fellowship for Schizophrenia and Related Disorders

http://www.world-schizophrenia.org/

The webpage of the World Fellowship for Schizophrenia and Related Disorders provides a general overview of disorders, information about current research, personal stories of individuals and families affected by the disorders, links to resources, and information about events happening around the world related to the disorders. This site may be useful to get a "global" view of the disorder in terms of better understanding it from the perspective of others around the world as well as getting an understanding of how impacted families and individuals are in other places of the world.

National Alliance on Mental Health

http://www.nami.org/Content/ContentGroups/Helpline1/Early_Onset_Schizophrenia.htm

The National Alliance on Mental Health advocates to ensure that all persons affected by mental illness receive the services that they need and deserve. This website provides a description of EOS, symptoms, diagnosis (as well as related difficulties), typical prognosis, common methods of treatment, common side effects of antipsychotic medications, and a brief overview of current research being conducted on EOS. Everything is explained in "layman's terms," making this website extremely user-friendly. It appears to be most geared toward families suspecting or living with affected children.

The American Academy of Child and Adolescent Psychiatry

http://www.aacap.org/cs/root/facts_for_families/schizophrenia_in_children

The American Academy of Child and Adolescent Psychiatry provides a brief primer for families interested in understanding schizophrenia in children. This site presents the common symptoms of EOS as well as some warning signs to be aware of in development. It also includes links to other psychiatric disorders (e.g., bipolar disorder and autism), to help families distinguish between commonly considered diagnoses that may precipitate or co-occur with the diagnosis of EOS.

The American Psychological Association

http://www.apa.org/topics/topicschiz.html

This page is the American Psychological Association's website dedicated to schizophrenia in general – not EOS specifically. However, as such, it includes information and links to resources that apply to children and their families. Specifically, it includes links to journals, books, other websites, and fact sheets.

Psychiatric Times

http://www.psychiatrictimes.com/schizophrenia

The Psychiatric Times website includes access to articles (e.g., research reviews, practice guidelines, clinical trials, and other news) that provides more information for individuals seeking further understanding of the etiology, epidemiology, assessment, and treatment of ECOS. Authored by medical professionals, this website includes information regarding differential diagnosis and comorbid diagnoses – rarely found on other sites. There are some articles specific to ECOS, including, "New Findings in Early-Onset Schizophrenia."

American Psychiatric Association
Americans with Disabilities Act of 1990 (ADA)
Americans with Disabilities Act Amendments Act (ADAAA)
Associated conditions
  Attention deficit hyperactivity disorder (ADHD)
  Atypical depression / dysthymic disorder
  Bipolar disorder
  Communication disorders
  Conduct disorder (CD)
  Learning disorders
  Major depressive disorder
  Obsessive-compulsive disorder (OCD)
  Oppositional defiant disorder (ODD)
  Pervasive developmental disorders (PDDs)
  Posttraumatic stress disorder (PTSD)
  Psychosis NOS
  Stereotypic movement disorder

- Brain abnormality
  - Hippocampus
  - Cortical gray matter
  - White matter
  - Ventricular ganglia
  - Basal ganglia
  - Superior temporal gyri
  - Hippocampal asymmetry
  - Larger ventricles
  - Smaller temporal lobes
  - Reduced metabolism in frontal lobe,
  - Significant reduction of mid sagittal thalamus
- Cognitive deficits
- Copy-number variations (CNVs)
- COS
- Depression
- *Diagnostic and Statistical Manual of Mental Disorders, Fourth Edition*
- *DSM IV-TR*
- Early onset schizophrenia
- Emotional Disturbance (ED)
- Environmental factors
  - Drug use
  - High latitude
  - Influenza
  - Inner city residence
  - Lead exposure
  - Natural disasters
  - Rubella
  - Vitamin D deficiency
  - Winter birth
- EOS symptoms
  - Achievement difficulties
  - Attention deficit
  - Delusions
  - Developmental delays
  - Disruptive behavior disorders
  - Hallucinations
  - Impaired memory and reasoning
  - Inappropriate or flattened expression of emotion
  - Isolation
  - Social withdrawal
  - Speech and language disorders
- Etiology
- Finnish Adoptive Family Study of Schizophrenia
- Incidence

Individualized Education Program (IEP)
Individuals with Disability Improvement Act (IDEIA, 2004)
Neurobiology
Prenatal /perinatal /postnatal risks
- Alpha-aminolevulinic acid
- Body mass index (BMI)
- Caesarean section
- Cigarette smoking
- Cytomegalovirus infections
- Delivery complications
- Labor-delivery complications (LDCs)
- Lead
- Loss of husband while pregnant
- Low birth weight
- Malnutrition
- Maternal hypertension
- Mumps
- Obstetric complications
- Toxins
- Viral infections

Prevalence
- Criminal/violent behaviors
- Developmental level
- Ethnicity
- Gender
- Migratory status
- Socioeconomic status (SES)
- Urbanization

Psychosis
Prodromal stage
Receptor genes
Rehabilitation Act of 1973
Section 504
Risk factors
- Child abuse
- Traumagenic neurodevelopmental (TN)
- Hippocampal damage
- Cerebral atrophy (loss of brain cells)
- Ventricular enlargement
- Reversed cerebral asymmetry

Risk genes
- Neuregulin
- Dysbindin
- D-amino acid oxidase
- Catechol-O-methyltransferase

- Proline dehydrogenase
- Reelin
- Serotonin type 2a receptor
- Dopamine D3 receptor

Schizoaffective disorder

Schizophrenia types

- Paranoid
- Disorganized
- Catatonic
- Undifferentiated
- Residual

Special education

Trauma

- Stigma
- Emotional abuse
- Physical abuse
- Sexual abuse
- Psychological abuse
- Neglect
- Bullying
- Bereavement/grief

References

Achenbach, T. (1998). Diagnosis, assessment, taxonomy, and case formulations. In T. Ollendick & M. Herson (Eds.), *Handbook of child psychopathology* (3rd ed., pp. 63–87). New York: Plenum Press.

Achenback, T. M., & Rescorla, L. A. (2001). Manual for the ASEBA school-age forms and profiles. Burlington, VT: University of Vermont, Research Center for Children, Youth, and Families.

Addington, J., Cadenhead, K.S., Cannon, T.D., Cornblatt, C., McGlashan, T., Perkins, D.O., & Heinssen, R. (2007). North American Prodrome Longitudinal Study: A collaborative multisite approach to prodromal schizophrenia research. *Schizophrenia Bulletin, 33*, 665–672.

Adelstein, A.M., Downham, D.Y., Stein, Z., & Susser, M.W. (1968). The epidemiology of mental illness in an English city: inceptions recognized by Salford Psychiatric services. *Social Psychiatry, 3*, 47–59.

Aesop Study Team (2002). Raised incidence of all psychosis in UK migrant populations. *Schizophrenia Research, 53*, 33.

Al Mousawi, A.H., & Dunstan, F.D. (1998). Changes in the risk of schizophrenia in Scotland: Is there an environmental factor? *Schizophrenia Bulletin, 24*, 529–535.

Alaghband-Rad, J., McKenna, K., Gordon, C.T., Albus, K. E., Hamburger, S.D., Rumsey, J. M., & Rapoport, J.L. (1995). Childhood onset schizophrenia: the severity of premorbid course. *Journal of the American Academy of Child and Adolescent Psychiatry, 34*, 1273–1283.

American Academy of Child and Adolescent Psychiatry (2001). Practice parameter for the assessment and treatment of children and adolescents with schizophrenia, *Journal of the American Academy of Child and Adolescent Psychiatry*, 40, 5s–23s.

American Psychiatric Association (2000). *Diagnostic and statistical manual of mental disorders* (4th ed., text rev.). Washington, DC: American Psychiatric Association.

Amminger, G.P., Leicester, S., Francey, S., & McGorry, P.D. (2005). The prodromal course. In R.L. Findling & S.C. Schulz (Eds.), *Juvenile Onset Schizophrenia: Assessment, Neurobiology, and Treatment*. (pp. 199–219). Baltimore, MD: John Hopkins Press.

Amminger, G.P., Paper, S., Rock, D., Roberts, S.A., Ott, S.L., & Squires-Kimling, I. (1999). Relationship between childhood behavioral disturbance and later schizophrenia in the New York High-Risk project. *American Journal of Psychiatry, 156*, 525–530.

Andreasen, N.C. (2000). Schizophrenia: The fundamental questions. *Brain Research Reviews, 31*, 106–112.

Armenteros, J.L., & Davies, M. (2006). Antipsychotics in early-onset schizophrenia: Systematic review and meta-analysis. *European Child and Adolescent Psychiatry, 15*, 14–148.

Armenteros, J.L., Whitaker, A.H., Welikson, M., Stedge, D.J., & Gorman, J. (1997). Risperdone in adolescents with schizophrenia: An open pilot study. *Journal of the American Academy of Child and Adolescent Psychiatry, 36*, 694–700.

Arseneault, L., Moffitt, T.E., Caspi, A., Taylor, P.J., & Silva, P.A. (2000). Mental disorders and violence in a total birth cohort: results from the Dunedin Study. *Archives of General Psychiatry, 57*, 979–968.

Asarnow, J.R., & Asarnow, R.F. (2003). Childhood-onset schizophrenia. In Mash, E.J., & Barkley, R.A. (Eds.), *Developmental psychopathology* (2nd ed., pp. 455–485). New York: Guilford Press.

Asarnow, R.F., Asamen, J., Granholm, E., Sherman, T., Watkins, J.M., & Williams, M.E. (1994). Cognitive/neuropsychological studies of children with a schizophrenic disorder. *Schizophrenia Bulletin, 20*, 647–669.

Asarnow, J.R., & Ben-Meir, S. (1988). Children with schizophrenia spectrum and depressive disorders: A comparative study of onset patterns, premorbid adjustment, and severity of dysfunction. *Journal of Child Psychology and Psychiatry, 29*, 477–488.

Asarnow, J.R., Thompson, M.C., & Goldstein, M.G. (1994). Childhood-onset schizophrenia: a follow-up study. *Schizophrenia Bulletin, 20*, 599–617.

Asarnow, J.R., Thompson, M.C., & McGrath, E.P. (2004). Annotation: Childhood-onset schizophrenia: Clinical and treatment issues. *Journal of Child Psychology and Psychiatry, 45*, 180–194.

Ayuso-Gutierrez, J.L., & del Rio, V. (1997). Factors influencing relapse in the long-term course of schizophrenia. *Schizophrenia Research, 28*, 199–206.

Badner, J.A., & Gershon, E.S. (2002). Meta-analysis of whole-genome linkage scans of bipolar disorder and schizophrenia. *Molecular Psychiatry, 7*, 405–411.

Bamrah, J.S., Freeman, H.L., & Goldberg, D.P. (1991). Epidemiology of schizophrenia in Salford, 1974–84. Changes in an urban community over ten years. *British Journal of Psychiatry, 159*, 802–810.

Bandura, A. (1977). *Social Learning Theory*. London: Prentice Hall.

Bellgrove, M.A., Vance, A., & Bradshaw, J.L. (2003). Local-global processing in early-onset schizophrenia: Evidence of an impairment in shifting the spatial scale of attention. *Brain and Cognition, 51*, 48–65.

Benton, M.K., & Schroeder, H.E. (1990). Social skills training with schizophrenics: A meta-analytic evaluation. *Journal of Consulting and Clinical Psychology, 58*, 741–747.

Bhugra, D., Hilwig, M., Hossein, B., Marceau, H., Neehall, J., Leff, J., & Der, G. (1996). First-contact incidence rates of schizophrenia in Trinidad and one-year follow-up. *British Journal of Psychiatry, 169*, 587–592.

Bhugra, D., Leff, J., Mallett, R., Der, G., Corridan, B. & Rudge, S. (1997). Incidence and outcome of schizophrenia in whites, African-Caribbeans and Asians in London. Psychological Medicine, *27*, 791–798.

Birchwood, M., Spencer, E., & McGovern, D. (2000). Schizophrenia: Early warning signs. *Advances in Psychiatry Treatment, 6*, 93–101.

Bland, R.C. (1977). Demographic aspects of functional psychoses in Canada. *Acta Psychiatrica Scandinavica, 55*, 369–80.

Bland, R.C. (1984). Long term mental illness in Canada: An epidemiological perspective on schizophrenia and affective disorders. *Canadian Journal of Psychiatry, 29*, 242–246.

Bland, R.C., & Orn, H. (1978). 14-year outcome in early schizophrenia. *Acta Psychiatrica Scandinavica, 58*, 327–338.

Blumenthal, J., Castellanos, F.X., Vaituzis, A.C., Fernandez, T., Hamburger, S.D., Liu, H., & Rapoport, J.L. (1999). Childhood-onset schizophrenia: Progressive brain changes during adolescence. *Biological Psychiatry, 46*, 892–898.

Bouras, N., Martin, G., Leese, M., Vanstraelen, M., Holt, G., Thomas, C., & Boardman, J. (2004). Schizophrenia-spectrum psychoses in people with and without intellectual disability. *Journal of Intellectual Disability Research, 48*(6), 548–555.

Boydell, J., & Murray, R. (2006). Urbanization, migration and risk of schizophrenia. In R.M. Murray, P. Jones, E. Susser, J. van Os, & M. Cannon (Eds.), *The Epidemiology of Schizophrenia* (pp.49–62). Cambridge, MA: The University Press.

Boydell, J., van Os, J., McKenzie, K., Allardyce, J., Goel, R., McCreadie, R.G., & Murray, R.M. (2001) Incidence of schizophrenia in ethnic minorities in London: Ecological study into interactions with environment. *British Medical Journal, 323*, 1336–1338.

Bradley, R., Henderson, K., & Monfore, D.A. (2004). A national perspective on children with emotional disorders. *Behavioral Disorders, 29*, 211–223.

Braw, Y., Bloch, Y., Medelovich, S., Ratzoni, G., Gal, G., Harari, H., & Levkovitz, Y. (2008). Cognition in young schizophrenia outpatients: Comparison of first-episode with multiepisode patients. *Schizophrenia Bulletin, 34*, 544–555.

Bromet, E.J., Dew, M.A., & Eaton, W. (1995). Epidemiology of psychosis with special reference to schizophrenia. In: Tsuang, M., Tohen, M., Zahner, G. (Eds.), *Textbook in Psychiatric Epidemiology* (pp. 283–300). New York: Wiley-Liss, Inc,.

Brown, A.S. (2006). Prenatal infection as a risk factor for schizophrenia. *Schizophrenia Bulletin*, 32(2), 200–202.

Brown, A.S. (2008). The risk for schizophrenia from childhood and adult infections. American Journal of Psychiatry *165*, 7–10.

Brown, R.T., Antonuccio, D.O., DuPaul, G.J., Fristad, M.A., King, C.A., Leslie, L.K., & Vitiello, B. (2008). Childhood mental health disorders: Evidence base and contextual factors for psychosocial, psychopharmacological, and combined interventions. Washington, DC: American Psychological Association.

Brown, A.S., Begg, M.D., Gravenstein, S., Schaefer, C.A., Wyatt, R.J., Bresnahan, M., & Susser E.S. (2004). Serologic evidence of prenatal influenza in the etiology of schizophrenia. *Archives of General Psychiatry*, *61*, 774–780.

Brown, A.S., Cohen, P., Haravy-Friedman, J., Babulas, V.S., Malaspina, D., Gorman, J., & Susser E.S. (2001). Prenatal rubella, premorbid abnormalities, and adult schizophrenia. *Biological Psychiatry*, *49*, 473–486.

Bruns, E (2008). The evidence base and wraparound. In E.J. Bruns & J.S. Walker (Eds.), *The resource guide to wraparound*. Portland, OR: National Wraparound Initiative, Research and Training Center for Family Support and Children's Mental Health.

Bryden, K.E., Carrey, N.J., & Kutcher, S.P. (2001). Update and recommendations for the use of antipsychotics in early-onset psychoses, *Journal of Child and Adolescent Psychopharmacology*, *11*, 113–130.

Buckley, P.F., Miller, B.J., Lehrer, D.S., & Castle, D.J. (2009). Psychiatric comorbidities and schizophrenia. *Schizophrenia Bulletin*, *35*, 383–402.

Burd, L. & Kerbeshian, J. (1987). A North Dakota prevalence study of schizophrenia presenting in childhood. *Journal of the American Academy of Child and Adolescent Psychiatry, 26*, 347–350.

Burke, L., Androutsos, C., Jogia, J., Byrne, P., & Frangou, S. (2008). The Maudsley early onset schizophrenia study: The effect of age of onset and illness duration on frontal-parietal gray matter. *European Psychiatry*, *23*, 233–236.

Burns, B.J., & Santos, A.B. (1995). Assertive community treatment: an update of randomized trials. *Psychiatric Services, 46*, 669–675.

Candilis, P.J. (2003). Early intervention in schizophrenia: Three frameworks for guiding ethical inquiry. *Psychopharmacology, 171*, 75–80.

Cannon, T.D., Cadenhead, K., Cornblatt, B., Woods, S.W., Addington, J., Walker, E., & Heinssen, R. (2008). Prediction of psychosis in youth at high clinical risk: A multisite longitudinal study in North America. *Archives of General Psychiatry*, *65*, 28–37.

Cannon, T.D., Rosso, I.M., Bearden, C.E., Sanchez, L.E., & Hadley, T. (1999). A prospective cohort study of neurodevelopmental processes in the genesis and epigenesis of schizophrenia. *Development and Psychopathology, 11*, 467–485.

Cantor-Graae, E., Pedersen, C.B., McNeil, T.F., & Mortensen, P.B. (2003). Migration as a risk factor for schizophrenia: A Danish population-based cohort study. *British Journal of Psychiatry, 182*, 117–122.

Caplan, R. (1994). Thought disorder in childhood. Journal of the *American Academy of Child and Adolescent Psychiatry*, 33, 605–615.

Cardno, A.G., Rijsdijk, F.V., Sham, P.C., Murray, R.M., & McGuffin, P. (2002). A twin study of genetic relationships between psychotic symptoms. *American Journal of Psychiatry*, 159, 539–545.

Carpenter, L., & Brockington, I.F. (1980). A study of mental illness in Asians, West Indians and Africans living in Manchester. British Journal of Psychiatry, 137, 201–205.

Carter, C.J. (2008). Schizophrenia susceptibility genes directly implicated in the life cycles of pathogens: Cytomegalovirus, influenza, herpes simplex, rubella, and *toxoplasma gondii*. *Schizophrenia Bulletin*, 35, 1163–1182.

Castle, D.J., & Murray, R.M. (1993). The epidemiology of late-onset schizophrenia. *Schizophrenia Bulletin, 19*, 691–700.

Castle, D.J., Wessely, S., Der, G., & Murray, R.M. (1991). The incidence of operationally defined schizophrenia in Camberwell, 1965–84. British Journal of Psychiatry, 159, 790–794.

Castro-Fornieles, J., Parellada, M., Soutullo, C.A., Baeza, I., Gonzalez-Pinto, A., Graell, M., & Arango, C. (2008). Antipsychotic treatment in child and adolescent first-episode psychosis: A longitudinal naturalistic approach. *Journal of Child and Adolescent Psychopharmacology, 18*, 327–336.

Cavanagh, J.T., & Shajahan, P.M. (1999). Increasing rates of hospital admission for men with major mental illnesses: data from Scottish mental health units, 1980–1995. *Acta Psychiatrica Scandinavica, 99*, 353–359.

Cervellione, K.L., Burdick, K.E., Cottone, J.G., Rhinewine, J.P., & Kumra, S. (2007). Neurocognitive deficits in adolescents with schizophrenia: longitudinal stability and predictive utility for short-term functional outcome. *Journal of the American Academy of Child and Adolescent Psychiatry, 46*, 867–878.

Chang, J., Golembo, S., Maeda, J., Tsuji, T., & Schiffman, J. (2008, September). *A psychometric analysis of five screening instruments for subthreshold symptoms of psychosis*. Paper presented at the Annual Conference of the Society for Research in Psychopathology. Pittsburgh, Pennsylvania.

Chen, C.H. (1984). Incidence and prevalence of schizophrenia in a community mental health service from 1975 to 1981. *Chinese Journal of Internal Medicine, 17*, 321–324.

Chowdhury, A.K. (1966). Admissions to an East Pakistan mental hospital. *British Journal of Psychiatry, 112*, 65–68.

Clark, A.F., & Lewis, S.W. (1998). Practitioner review: Treatment of schizophrenia in childhood and adolescence, *Journal of Child Psychology and Psychiatry*, 39, 1071–1081.

Cochrane, R., & Bal, S.S. (1987). Migration and schizophrenia: an examination of five hypotheses. *Social Psychiatry*, 22, 181–191.

Cochrane, R., & Bal, S.S. (1989). Mental hospital admission rates of immigrants to England: A comparison of 1971 and 1981. *Social Psychiatry and Psychiatric Epidemiology*, 24, 2–11.

Coid, J.W., Kirkbride, J.B., Barker, D., Cowden, F., Stamps, R., Yang, M., & Jones, P.B.. (2008). Raised incidence rates of all psychoses among migrant groups: findings from the East London first episode psyhosis study. *Archives of General Psychiatry, 65*(11), 1250–1258.

Coleman, R. (1973). A procedure for fading from experimenter-school based to parent-home based control of classroom behavior. *Journal of School Psychology, 11*, 71–79.

Corcoran, C., Davidson, L., Sills-Shahar, R., Nickou, C., Malaspina, D., Miller, T., & McGlashan, T. (2003). A qualitative research study of the evolution of symptoms in individuals identified as prodromal to psychosis. *Psychiatry Quarterly*, 74, 313–332.

Cornblatt, B., Lencz, T., & Kane, J.M. (2001). Treatment of schizophrenia prodrome: Is it presently ethical? *Schizophrenia Research, 51*, 31–38.

Cornblatt, B., Lencz, T., & Obuchowski, M. (2002). The schizophrenia prodrome: Treatment and high risk perspective. *Schizophrenia Research, 54*, 177–186.

Cornblatt, B., Obuchowski, M., Roberts, S., Pollack, S., & Erlenmeyer-Kimling, L. (1999). Cognitive and behavioral precursors of schizophrenia. *Development and Psychopathology, 11*, 487–508.

Craddock, N., O'Donovan, M.C., & Owen, M. J. (2006). Genes for schizophrenia and bipolar disorder? Implications for psychiatric nosology. *Schizophrenia Bulletin*, 32, 9–16.

Dalman, C., Allebeck, P., Gunnell, D., Harrison, G., Kristensson, K., Lewis, G., & Karlsson, H (2008). Infections in the CNS during childhood and the risk of subsequent psychotic illness: A cohort study of more than one million Swedish subjects. *American Journal of Psychiatry*, 165, 59–65.

D'Arcy, C., Rawson, N.S.B., Lydick E., & Epstein R. (1993). The epidemiology of treated schizophrenia Saskatchewan 1976–1990. *In World Psychiatric Association, Section of Epidemiology and Community Psychiatry. The Netherlands* 1993.

Davila, R.R., Williams, M.L., & MacDonald, J.T. (1991, September 16). *Memorandum to chief state school officers re: Clarification of policy to address the needs of children with attention deficit disorders with general and/or special education.* Washington, DC: U.S. Department of Education.

Davidson, M., Reichenberg, A., Rabinowitz, J., Weiser, M., Kaplan, Z., & Mark, M. (1999). Behavioral and intellectual markers for schizophrenia in apparently healthy male adolescents. *American Journal of Psychiatry* 156, 1328–1335.

Davidson, L., Stayner, D., & Haglund, K.E. (1998). Phenomological perspectives on the social functioning of people with schizophrenia. In K.T. Mueser & N. Tarrier (Eds.), *Handbook of Social Functioning in Schizophrenia* (pp.97–120). Needham Heights, MA: Allyn and Bacon.

De Alarcon, J.G., & Seagroatt, V. (1990). Trends in schizophrenia. *Lancet, 335*, 852–853.

De Salvia, D., Barbato, A., Salvo, P., & Zadro, F. (1993). Prevalence and incidence of schizophrenic disorders in Portogruaro: An Italian case register study. *Journal of Nervous Mental Disorder, 181*, 275–82.

Dean, G., Downing, H., & Shelley, E. (1981). First admissions to psychiatric hospitals in south-east England in 1976 among immigrants from Ireland. *British Medical Journal (Clinical Research Edition)*, 282, 1831–1833.

Dean, G., Walsh, D., Downing, H., & Shelley, E. (1981). First admissions of native-born and immigrants to psychiatric hospitals in South-East England 1976. *British Journal of Psychiatry*, 139, 506–512.

Delisi, L.E. (1992). The significance of age of onset for schizophrenia. *Schizophrenia. Bulletin*, 18, 209–215.

Delis, D.C., Kramer, J.H., Kaplan, E., & Ober, B.A. (1987). *California Verbal Learning Test.* San Antonio, TX: Pearson.

Der, G., Gupta, S., & Murray, R.M. (1990). Is schizophrenia disappearing? *Lancet, 335*, 513–516.

Dickerson, F.B. (2000). Cognitive behavioral psychotherapy for schizophrenia: A review of recent empirical studies. *Schizophrenia Research, 16*, 71–90.

Dickerson, F.B., Tenhula, W.N., & Green-Paden, L.D. (2005). The token economy for schizophrenia: Review of the literature and recommendations for future research. *Schizophrenia Research, 75*, 405–416.

Dilk, M.N., & Bond, G.R. (1996). Meta-analytic evaluation of skills training research for individuals with severe mental illness: Review of recent studies. *Journal of Consulting and Clinical Psychology, 64*, 1337–346.

Dixon, L.B., Lehman, A.F., & Levine, J. (1995). Conventional antipsychotic medications for schizophrenia. *Schizophrenia Bulletin, 4*, 567–577.

Doane, J.A., Goldstein, M.J., Miklowitz, D.J., & Falloon, I.R.H. (1986). The impact of individual and family treatment on the affective climate of families of schizophrenics. *British Journal of Psychiatry, 148*, 279–287.

Doody, G.A., Johnstone, E.C., Sanderson, T.L., Owens D.G., & Muir W.J. (1998). 'Pfropfschizophrenie' revisited: Schizophrenia in people with mild learning disability. *British Journal of Psychiatry*, 173, 145–153.

Dougherty, E.H., & Schinka, J.A. (1989). *Mental status checklist for adolescents.* Lutz, FL: Psychological Assessment Resources, Inc.

Downing, D., & Spring, E. (2007). Community collaboration helps to target early detection and intervention for psychosis. *National Council Magazine, 3*, 32–33.

Drasgow, E., & Yell, M.L. (2001). Functional behavioral assessments: Legal requirements and challenges. *School Psychology Review, 20*, 239–251.

Drury, B., Birchwood, M., & Cochrane, R. (2000).Cognitive therapy and recovery form acute psychosis: A controlled trial III. Five-year follow-up. *British Journal of Psychiatry, 177*, 8–14.

Dulmus, C.N., & Smyth, N.J. (2000). Early-onset schizophrenia: A literature review of empirically based interventions. *Child and Adolescent Social Work Journal*, 17, 55–69.

Dunham, H.W. (1965). *Community and Schizophrenia: an epidemiological analysis* Detroit, Michigan: Wayne State University Press 1965.

Eagles, J.M., Hunter, D., & McCance, C. (1988). Decline in the diagnosis of schizophrenia among first contacts with psychiatric services in north-east Scotland, 1969–1984. *British Journal of Psychiatry, 152*, 793–798.

Eagles, J.M., & Whalley, L.J. (1985). Decline in the diagnosis of schizophrenia among first admissions to Scottish mental hospitals from 1969–78. *British Journal of Psychiatry, 146*, 151–154.

Eastvold, A.D., Heaton, R.K., & Cadenhead, K.S. (2007). Neurocognitive deficits in the (putative) prodrome and first episode of psychosis. *Schizophrenia Research, 93*, 266–277.

Eaton, W.W. (1974). Residence, social class, and schizophrenia. *Journal of Health and Social Behavior, 15*, 289–299.

Eaton, W.W., & Levav, I. (1982). Schizophrenia, social class and ethnic disadvantage. A study of first hospitalization among Israeli-born Jews. *The Israel Journal of Psychiatry and related sciences, 19*(4), 289–302.

Eber, L., Sugai, G., Smith, C.R., & Scott, T.M. (2002). Wraparound and positive behavioral interventions and supports in the schools. *Journal of Emotional and Behavioral Disorders, 10*, 171–180.

Eggers, C., & Bunk, D. (1997). The long-term course of childhood-onset schizophrenia: A 42 year followup. *Schizophrenia Bulletin*, 23, 105–117.

Eggers, C., Bunk, D., & Krause, D. (2000). Schizophrenia with onset before the age of eleven: Clinical characteristics of onset and course. *Journal of Autism and Developmental Disorders*, 30, 29–38.

Erhart, S.M., Marder, S.R., & Carpenter, W.T. (2006). Treatment of schizophrenia negative symptoms: Future prospects. *Schizophrenia Bulletin, 32*, 234–237.

Eronen, M., Hakola, P., & Tiihonen, J. (1996). Mental disorders and homicidal behavior in Finland. *Archives of General Psychiatry, 53*, 497–501.

Fagerlund, B., Pagsberg, A.K., & Hemmingsen, R.P. (2006). Cognitive deficits and levels of IQ in adolescent onset schizophrenia and other psychotic disorders. *Schizophrenia Research, 85*, 30–39.

Faris, R., & Dunham, H. (1939). *Mental Disorders in Urban Areas*. Chicago, IL: University of Chicago Press.

Fatemi, S.H., & Folsom, T.D. (2009). The neurodevelopmetnal hypothesis of schizophrenia, revisited. *Schizophrenia Bulletin*, 35, 528–548.

Fearon, P., Kirkbride, J.B., Morgan, C., Dazzan, P., Morgan, K., & Lloyd, T., et al. (2006). Incidence of schizophrenia and other psychoses in ethnic minority groups: results from the MRC AESOP Study. *Psychological Medicine, 36*(11), 1541–1550.

Fenton, W.S., Blyler, C.R., & Heinssen, R.K., (1997). Determinants of medication compliance in schizophrenia: Empirical and clinical findings. *Schizophrenia Bulletin, 23*, 637–651.

Fields, J.H., Grochowski, S., Lindenmayer, J.P., Kay, S.R., Grosz, D., & Hyman R.B., et al. (1994). Assessing positive and negative symptoms in children and adolescents. *American Journal of Psychiatry*, 151, 249–253.

Findling, R.L., Robb, A., Nyilas, M., Forbes, R.A., Jin, N., & Ivanova, S., et al. (2008). A multiple-center, randomized, double-blind, placebo-controlled study of oral aripiprazole for treatment of adolescents with schizophrenia. *American Journal of Psychiatry, 165*, 1432–1441.

Findling, R.L., & Schulz, S.C. (2005). *Juvenile-Onset Schizophrenia: Assessment, Neurobiology, and Treatment*. Baltimore, MD: John Hopkins Press.

Fish, B., Marcus, J., Hans, S.L., Auerbach, J.G., & Perdue, S. (1992). Infants at risk for schizophrenia: Sequelae of a genetic neurointegrative deficit. A review and replication analysis of pandysmaturation in the Jerusalem Infant Development Study. *Archives of General Psychiatry, 49*, 221–235.

Fleishhaker, C., Schulz, E., Tepper, K., Martin, M., Hennighausen, K., & Remschmidt, H. (2005). Long-term course of adolescent schizophrenia. *Schizophrenia Bulletin, 31*, 1–12.

Folnegovic, Z., Folnegovic-Smalc, V., & Kulcar, Z. (1990). The incidence of schizophrenia in Croatia. *British Journal of Psychiatry, 156*, 363–365.

Fontaine, K.L. (2009). *Mental Health Nursing: Sixth Edition*. Upper Saddle River, NJ: Prentice Hall.

Frazier, F.A., McClellan, J., Findling, R.L., Vitiello, B., Anderson, R., Zablotsky, B., et al. (2007). Treatment of early-onset schizophrenia spectrum disorders (TEOSS): Demographic and clinical characteristics. *Journal of American Academy of Child and Adolescent Psychiatry, 46*, 979–988.

Fuller, R., Nopoulos, P., Arndt, S., O'Leary, D., Ho, B.C., & Andreasen, N.C., (2002). Longitudinal assessment of premorbid cognitive functioning in patients with schizophrenia through examination of standardized scholastic test performance. *American Journal of Psychiatry, 159*, 1183–1189.

Garety, P.A., Fowler, D., & Kuipers, E. (2000). Cognitive-behavioral therapy for medication-resistant symptoms. *Schizophrenia Bulletin, 26*, 73–86.

Garety, P.A., & Freeman, D. (1999). Cognitive approaches to delusions: A critical review of theories and evidence. *British Journal of Clinical Psychology, 38*, 113–154.

Geddes, J.R., Black, R.J., Whalley, L.J., & Eagles, J.M. (1993). Persistence of the decline in the diagnosis of schizophrenia among first admissions to Scottish hospitals from 1969 to 1988. *British Journal of Psychiatry, 163*, 620–626.

Geddes, J. R., & Lawrie, S. M. (1995). Obstetric complications and schizophrenia: A meta-analysis. *British Journal of Psychiatry, 167*, 786–793.

Giedd, J.N., Jeffries, N.O., Blumenthal, J., Castellanos, F.X., Vaituzis, A.C., Fernandez, T., Hamburgera, S.D., Liua, H., Nelsona, J., Bedwella, J., Trana, L., Lenanea, M., Nicolsona, R., & Rapoport, J.L. (1999). Childhood-onset schizophrenia: Progressive brain changes during adolescence. Biological Psychiatry, *46*, 892–898.

Giel, R., Sauer, H.C., Slooff, C.J., & Wiersma, D. (1980). Over de epidemiologie van functionele psychosen en invaliditeit [Epidemiological observations on schizophrenia and disability in the Netherlands]. *Tijdschrift voor psychiatrie, 22*, 710–722

Giggs, J. (1973). High rates of schizophrenia among immigrants in Nottingham. *Nursing Times, 69*, 1210–1212.

Gillberg, C., Hellgren, L., & Gillberg, C. (1993). Psychotic disorders diagnosed in adolescence. Outcome at age 30 years. *Journal of Child Psychology and Psychiatry and Allied Disciplines, 34*, 1173–1185.

Gioia, D., & Brekke, J. S. (2003). Rehab rounds: Use of the Americans with Disabilities Act by young adults with Schizophrenia. *Psychiatry Services, 54*, 302–304.

Goater, N., King, M., Cole, E., Leavey, G., Johnson-Sabine, E., & Blizard, R., et al. (1999). Ethnicity and outcome of psychosis. *British Journal of Psychiatry, 175*, 34–42.

Gochman, P.A., Greenstein, D., Sporn, A., Gogtay, N., & Keller, B., et al. (2005). IQ stabilization in childhood-onset schizophrenia. *Schizophrenia Research, 77*, 271–277.

Gogtay, N. (2008). Cortical brain development in schizophrenia: Insights from neuroimaging studies in childhood-onset schizophrenia. *Schizophrenia Bulletin, 34*, 30–36.

Gale, G., Pfefferbaum, B., Suhr, M.A., & Overall, J.E. (1986). The Brief Psychiatric Rating Scales for Children; A reliability study. *Journal of Clinical Child & Adolescent Psychology*, 15, 341–345.

Gogtay N., Sporn, A., Clasen, L.S., Greenstein, D., Giedd, G.N., & Lenane, M., et al. (2003). Structural brain MRI abnormalities in healthy siblings of patients with childhood-onset schizophrenia. *American Journal of Psychiatry, 160*, 569–571.

Goldacre, M., Shiwach, R., & Yeates, D. (1994). Estimating incidence and prevalence of treated psychiatric disorders from routine statistics: the example of schizophrenia in Oxfordshire. *Journal of Epidemiological Community Health, 48*, 318–322.

Goldstein, M.J., & Miklowitz, D.J. (1995). The effectiveness of psychoeducational family therapy in the treatment of schizophrenic disorders. *Journal of Marital and Family Therapy, 21*, 361–376.

Gonthier, M., & Lyon, M.A. (2004). Childhood-onset schizophrenia: An overview. *Psychology in the Schools, 41*, 803–811.

Gourovitch, M.L., Goldberg, T.E., & Weinberger, D.R. (1996). Verbal fluency deficits in patients with schizophrenia: semantic fluency is differentially impaired as compared with phonological fluency. *Neuropsychology 10*, 573–577.

Grawe, R., Levander, S., & Krueger, M. (1991). Incidence, clinical characteristics, and short-term outcome of first-episode schizophrenia. *Nordisk Psykiatrisk Tidsskrift, 45*, 383–390.

Green, M.F., Kern, R.S., Braff, D.L., & Mintz, J. (2000). Neurocognitive deficits and functional outcome in schizophrenia: Are we measuring the "right stuff"? *Schizophrenia Bulletin, 26*, 119–136.

Gresham, F., & Elliott, S. (1990). *Social Skills Rating Scale*. Circle Pines, MN: American Guidance Services.

Gross, G., Huber, G., Klosterkötter, J., & Linz, M. (1987). *BSABS: Bonn Scale for the Assessment of Basic Symptoms*. Berlin: Springer.

Hafner, H., & An der Heiden, W. (1986). The contribution of European case registers to research on schizophrenia. *Schizophrenia Bulletin, 12*, 26–51.

Hafner, H., & Maurer, K. (2006). Early detection of schizophrenia: Current evidence and future perspectives. *World Psychiatry, 5*, 130–138.

Hafner, H., Maurer, K., Trendler, G., an der Heiden, W., Schmidt, M., & Konnecke, R. (2005). Schizophrenia and depression: Challenging the paradigm of two separate diseases–a controlled study of schizophrenia, depression, and healthy controls. *Schizophrenia Research, 77*, 11–24.

Hans, S.L., & Marcus, J. (1991). Neurobehavioral development of infants at risk for schizophrenia: A review. In Walker, E.F. (ed.) *Schizophrenia: A life-course developmental perspective*. New York: Academic Press.

Harrison, G. (1990). Searching for the causes of schizophrenia: The role of migrant studies. *Schizophrenia Bulletin, 16*, 663–671.

Harrison, G., Cooper, J.E., & Gancarczyk, R. (1991). Changes in the administrative incidence of schizophrenia. *British Journal of Psychiatry, 159*, 811–816.

Harrison, G., Glazebrook, C., Brewin, J., Cantwell, R., Dalkin, T., & Fox, R., et al. (1997). Increased incidence of psychotic disorders in migrants from the Caribbean to the United Kingdom. *Psychological Medicine*, 27, 799–806.

Harrison, G., Owens, D., Holton, A., Neilson, D. & Boot, D. (1988). A prospective study of severe mental disorder in Afro-Caribbean patients. *Psychological Medicine, 18*, 643–657.

Hata, K., Iida, J., Iwasaka, H., Negoro, H.I., Ueda, F., & Kishimoto, T. (2003). Minor physical anomalies in childhood and adolescent onset schizophrenia. *Psychiatry and Clinical Neurosciences, 57*, 17–21.

Haugaard, J.J. (2004). Recognizing and treating rare behavioral and emotional disorders in children and adolescents who have been severely maltreated: Schizophrenia. *Child Maltreatment, 9*, 161–168.

Heinimaa, M., Salokangas, R., Ristkari, T., Plathin, M., Huttunen, J., & Ilonen, T., et al. (2003). PROD-screen–a screen for prodromal symptoms of psychosis. *International Journal of Methods in Psychiatric Research, 12*, 92–104.

Helgason, L. (1977). Psychiatric services and mental illness in Iceland. Incidence study (1966–1967) with 6–7 year follow-up. *Acta Psychiatrica Scandinavica Supplement, 1*–140.

Hemsi, L.K. (1967). Psychiatric morbidity of West Indian immigrants. *Social Psychiatry, 2*, 95–100.

Henquet, C., Krabbendam, L., Dautzenberg, J., Jolles, J., & Merckelback, H. (2005). Confusing thoughts and speech: Source monitoring and psychosis. *Psychiatry Research*, 133, 57–63.

Hickling, F.W., Rodgers-Johnson, P. (1995). The incidence of first contact schizophrenia in Jamaica. *British Journal of Psychiatry, 167*, 193–196.

Hitch, P.J., & Rack, P.H. (1980). Mental illness among Polish and Russian refugees in Bradford. *British Journal of Psychiatry*, 137, 206–211.

Ho, B., Andreasen, N., Nopoulos, P., Fuller, R., Arndt, S., & Cadoret, R.J. (2005). Secondary prevention of schizophrenia: Utility of standardized scholastic tests for early identification. *Annals of Clinical Psychiatry, 17*, 11–18.

Hogarty, G.E. (2002). Personal therapy: A practical psychotherapy for stabilization of schizophrenia. In S.G. Hoffman & M.C. Tompson (Eds.), *Treating Chronic and Severe Mental Disorders: A Handbook of Empirically-Supported Interventions*. New York: Guilford Press.

Hogarty, G.E., & Ulrich, R.F. (1998). The limitations of antipsychotic medications on schizophrenia relapse and adjustment and the contributions of psychosocial treatment. *Journal of Psychiatric Research, 32*, 243–250.

Hollis, C. (1995). Child and adolescent (juvenile onset) schizophrenia. A case control study of premorbid development impairments. *British Journal of Psychiatry, 166*, 489–495.

Hollis, C. (2003). Developmental precursors of child-and adolescent-onset schizophrenia and affective psychoses: diagnostic specificity and continuity with symptom dimensions. *British Journal of Psychiatry, 182*, 37–44.

House, A.E. (1999). *DSM-IV diagnosis in the schools*. New York: The Guilford Press.

Howes, O.D., & Kapur, S. (2009). The dopamine hypothesis of schizophrenia: Version III- The final common pathway. *Schizophrenia Bulletin, 35*, 549–562.

Iacono, W.G., & Beiser, M. (1992). Are males more likely than females to develop schizophrenia? *American Journal of Psychiatry, 149*, 1070–1074.

Jablensky, A., Sartorius, N., Ernberg, G., Anker, M., Korten, A., & Cooper, J.E., et al. (1992). Schizophrenia: manifestations, incidence and course in different cultures. A World Health Organization ten-country study. *Psychological Medicine Monograph Supplement, 20*, 1–97.

James, D., Mukherjee, T., & Smith, C. (1996). Schizophrenia and learning disability. *British Journal of Learning Disabilities, 24*(3), 90–94.

Johannessen, J.O. (1985). Schizofreni-forekomst i et norsk fylke, Rogaland. *Nord Psykiatr Tidsskr, 39*, 217–223.

Jones, P., Rodgers, B., Murray, R., & Marmot, M. (1994). Child development risk factors for adult schizophrenia in the British 1946 birth cohort. *Lancet, 344*,1398–1402.

Jorgensen, P. (1986). Delusional psychosis : Hospital incidence, symptoms and classification. *Acta Psychiatrica Scandinavica, 74*, 18–23.

Joyce, P.R. (1987). Changing trends in first admissions and readmissions for mania and schizophrenia in New Zealand, 1974 to 1984. *Australian and New Zealand Journal of Psychiatry, 21*, 82–86.

Karson, C., & Bigelow, L.B. (1987). Violent behaviour in schizophrenia patients. *Journal of Nervous and Mental Diseases, 175*, 161–164.

Kaufman, J., Birmaher, B., Brent, D., Rao, U., Flynn, C., & Moreci, P., et al (1997). Schedule for affective disorders and schizophrenia for school-age children –present and lifetime version (KSADS-PL): initial reliability and validity data. *Journal of the American Academy of Child and Adolescent Psychiatry*, 36,980–8.

Kaufman, J., Birmaher, B., Brent, D., Rao, U., & Ryan, N. (1996). *The schedule for affective disorders and schizophrenia for school-age children*. Pittsburgh: University of Pittsburgh Medical Center.

Kazdin, A.E., & Bootzin, R.R. (1972). The token economy: An evaluative review. *Journal of Applied Behavioral Analysis, 5*, 343–372.

Keith, S.J., Reiger, D.A., & Rae, D.S. (1991). Schizophrenic disorders. In: L.N. Robbins & D.A. Reiger, (Eds.), *Psychiatric Disorders in America* (pp.33–52). New York, NY: The Free Press.

Kelsey, J.E., Newport, D.J., & Nemeroff, C. B. (2006). *Principles of Psychopharmacology for Mental Health Professionals*. John Wiley & Sons, Inc.

Kendell, R.E., Malcolm, D.E., & Adams, W. (1993). The problem of detecting changes in the incidence of schizophrenia. *British Journal of Psychiatry, 162*, 212–218.

Kendler, K.S., Gallagher, T.J., Abelson, J.M., & Kessler, R.C. (1996). Lifetime prevalence, demographic risk factors, and diagnostic validity of nonaffective psychosis as assessed in a US community sample: The National Comorbidity Survey. Archives of General Psychiatry, *53*, 1022–1031.

Kendziora, K., Bruns, E., Osher, D., Pacchiano, D., & Mejia, B. (2001). *Systems of Care: Promising Practices in Children's Mental Health, 2001 Series, Volume 1*. Washington, D.C.: Center for Effective Collaboration and Practice, American Institutes for Research.

Kenny, J.R., Friedman, L., Findling, R.L., Swales, T.P., Strauss, M.E., Jesberger, J.A., & Schulz, S.C. (1997). Cognitive impairment in adolescents with schizophrenia. *American Journal of Psychiatry, 154*, 1613–1615.

King, M.E., Coker, M., Leavey, G., Hoare, A. & Johnson-Sabine, E. (1994). Incidence of psychotic illness in London: comparison of ethnic groups. *British Medical Journal, 309*, 1115–1119.

Kinney, D.K., Teixeira, P., Hsu, D., Napoleon, S.C., Crowley, D.J., & Miller, A., et al. (2009). Relation of schizophrenia prevalence to latitude, climate, fish consumption, infant mortality, and skin color: A role for prenatal Vitamin D deficiency and infections? *Schizophrenia Bulletin, 35*, 568–576.

Kirkbride, J.B., Barker, D., Cowden, F., Stamps, R., Yang, J., & Jones, P.B. et al. (2008). Psychoses, ethnicity and socio-economic status. *British Journal of Psychiatry, 193*(1), 18–24.

Kline, R.B., Lachar D., & Sprague, D.J. (1985). The Personality Inventory for Children (PIC): An Unbiased Predictor of Cognitive and Academic Status. *Journal of Pediatric Psychology, 10*, 461–477.

Kirkbride, J.B., Boydell, J., Ploubidis, G.B., Morgan, C., Dazzan, P., & McKenzie, K., et al. (2008). Testing the association of incidence of schizophrenia and social capital in an urban area. *Psychological Medicine, 38*(8), 1083–1094.

Kline, R.B., Lachar, D., & Sprague, D. (1985). The Personality Inventory for Children (PIC): An unbiased predictor of cognitive and academic status. *Journal of Pediatric Psychology, 10*, 461–477.

Klosterkotter, J., Hellmich, M., Steinmeyer, E.M., & Schultze-Lutter, F. (2001). Diagnosing schizophrenia in the initial prodrome phase. *Archives of General Psychiatry, 58*, 158–164.

Kodish, I., & McClellan, J. (2007). Early-onset schizophrenia. In M. Hersen & D. Reitman, *Handbook of psychological assessment, case conceptualization, and treatment, Vol 2: Children and adolescents* (pp. 405–443). Hoboken, NJ, US: John Wiley & Sons Inc.

Kolvin, C., Ounsted, M., Humphrey, M., & McNay, A. (1971). The phenomenology of childhood psychoses. *British Journal of Psychiatry, 118*, 385–395.

Kranzler, H., Roofeh, D., Gerbino-Rosen, G., Dombrowski, C., McMeniman, M., & DeThomas, C., et al. (2005). Clozapine: Its impact on aggressive behavior among children and adolescents with schizophrenia. *Journal of the American Academy of Child and Adolescent Psychiatry, 44*, 55–63.

Kravariti, E., Morris, R.G., Rabe-Hesketh, S., Murray, R., & Frangou, S. (2003). The Maudsley early-onset schizophrenia study: Cognitive function in adolescent- onset schizophrenia. *Schizophrenia Research, 65*, 95–103.

Kronenberger, W.G., & Meyer, R.G. (2001). *The Child Clinician's Handbook (Second Edition)*. Boston: Allyn and Bacon.

Krupinski, J., & Cochrane, R. (1980). Migration and mental health –a comparative study. *Journal of International Studies, 1*, 49–57.

Kumra, S., Nicolson, R., & Rapoport, J.L. (2002). Childhood-onset schizophrenia: Research update. In R. B. Zipursky & S. C. Schulz (Eds.). *The early stages of schizophrenia* (pp. 161–190). Washington, D.C.: American Psychiatric Publishing, Inc.

Kumra, S., & Schulz, S.C. (2008). Editorial: Research progress in Early-Onset Schizophrenia. *Schizophrenia Bulletin, 34* (1), 15–17.

Kuusi, K. (1986). Prognosis of schizophrenia psychosis in Helsinki in 1975–1983. *Monographs of Psychiatria Fennica, 13*.

Lachar, D., & Gruber, O. P. (1995). *Personality Inventory for Youth (PIY) manual Administration and interpretation guide*. Los Angeles: Western Psychological Services.

Lachar, D., Randle, S.L., Harper R.A., Scott-Gurnell, K.C., & Lewis, K.R., & Santos, C.W et al. (2001). The Brief Psychiatric Rating Scale for Children (BPRS-C): Validity and reliability of an anchored version. *Journal of American Academy Child and Adolescent Psychiatry, 40*, 333–340.

Larsen, T.K., Friis, S., Haahr, U., Joa, I., Johannessen, J.O., Melle, I., & Vaglum, P (2001). Early detection and intervention in first-episode schizophrenia: A critical review. *Acta Psychiatrica Scandinavica, 103*, 323–334.

Lawrie, S.M., & Abukmeil, S.S. (1998). Brain abnormality in schizophrenia: A systematic and quantitative review of volumetric magnetic resonance imaging studies. *British Journal of Psychiatry, 172*, 110–120.

Lawrie, S.M., McIntosh, A.M., Hall, J., Owens, D.G., & Johnstone, E.C. (2008). Brain structure and function changes during the development of schizophrenia: The evidence from studies of subjects at increased genetic risk. *Schizophrenia Bulletin, 34*, 330–40.

Lay, B., Blanz, B., Hartmann, M., & Schmidt, M.H. (2000). The psychosocial outcome of adolescent-onset schizophrenia: A 12-year followup. *Schizophrenia Bulletin, 26*(4), 801–816.

Lee, F., McGlashan, T.H., & Woods, S.W. (2005). Prevention of schizophrenia: Can it be achieved? *CNS Drugs, 19*, 193–206.

Lehman, A.F., Kreyenbuhl, J., Buchanan, R.W., Dickerson, F.B., Dixon, L.B., Goldberg, R., & Steinwachs, D.M. (2004). The Schizophrenia Patient Outcomes Research Team (PORT): Updated treatment recommendations 2003. *Schizophrenia Bulletin, 30*, 193–217.

Lehtinen, V., Veijola, J., Lindholm, T., Moring, J., Puukka, P., & Vaisanen, E. (1996). Incidence of mental disorders in the Finnish UKKI study. *British Journal of Psychiatry, 168*, 672–678.

Lewis, G., David, A., Andreasson, S., & Allebeck, P. (1992). Schizophrenia and city life. *Lancet, 340*, 137–140.

Lewis, D.A., & Levitt, P. (2002). Schizophrenia as a disorder of neurodevelopment. *Annual Review of Neuroscience, 25*, 409–432.

Li, H. (2004). *Fears and related anxieties in children having a disability*. Dissertation Abstracts International Section A: Humanities and Social Sciences Vol 64(9-A), 3190.

Lieberman, J.A., Perkins, D., Belger, A., Chakos, M., Jarskog, F., Boteva, K., & Gilmore, J. (2001). The early stages of schizophrenia: Speculations on pathogenesis, pathophysiology, and therapeutic approaches. *Biological Psychiatry, 50*, 884–897.

Lieberman, Y.I. (1974). The incidence of schizophrenia (materials from a clinico-epidemiologic study). *Zhurnal nevropatologii i psikhiatrii imeni S.S. Korsakova, 74*, 1224–1233.

Lindamer, L.A., Lohr, J.B., Harris, M.J., & Jeste, D.V. (2004). Gender, Estrogen, and Schizophrenia. *American Psychiatric Association*, 2, 138–145.

Loewy, R.L., Bearden, C.E., Johnson, J.K., Raine, A., & Cannon, T.D. (2005). The prodromal questionnaire (PQ): Preliminary validation of a self-report screening measure for prodromal and psychotic syndromes. *Schizophrenia Research, 79*, 117–125.

Loewy, R.L. & Cannon, T.D. (2008). The Prodromal Questionnaire- Brief Version (PQ-B). University of California.

Loffler, W., & Hafner, H. (1999). Ecological pattern of first admitted schizophrenics in two German cities over 25 years. *Social Science & Medicine, 49*, 93–108.

Lynge, I., & Jacobsen, J. (1995). Schizophrenia in Greenland: A follow-up study. *Acta Psychiatrica Scandinavica, 91*, 414–422.

Lynge, I., Mortensen, P.B., & Munk-Jorgensen, P. (1999). Mental disorders in the Greenlandic population: A register study. *International Journal of Circumpolar Health, 58*, 188–197.

Lupski, J.R. (2008). Schizophrenia: Incriminating genomic evidence. *Nature 455*, 178–179.

Ma, S.P. (1980). An epidemiologic investigation of psychoses in Laoshan County of Qingdao. *Chinese Journal of Internal Medicine, 13*, 22–23.

MacCabe, J.H.., Lambe, M.P., Cnattingius, S., Torrang, A., Bjork, C., Sham, P.C., & Hultman, C.M. (2008). Scholastic achievement at age 16 and risk of schizophrenia and other psychoses: A national cohort study. *Psychological Medicine, 38*, 1133–1140.

McGrath, J., Saha, S., Welham, J., El Saadi, O., MacCauley, C., & Chant, D. (2004). A systematic review of the incidence of schizophrenia: the distribution of rates and the influence of sex, urbanicity, migrant status and methodology. BMC Medicine, 2 (13), 1-22. doi:10.1186/1741-7015-2-13

Mahy, G.E., Mallett, R., Leff, J., & Bhugra, D. (1999). First-contact incidence rate of schizophrenia on Barbados. *British Journal of Psychiatry, 175*, 28–33.

Malaspina, D., Goetz, R.R., Yale, S., Berman, A., Friedman, J.H., Tremeau, F., & Gorman, J.M. (2000). Relation of familial schizophrenia to negative symptoms but not to the deficit syndrome. *American Journal of Psychiatry, 157*, 994–1003.

Malmberg, A., Lewis, G., David, A., & Allebeck, P. (1998). Premorbid adjustment and personality in people with schizophrenia. *British Journal of Psychiatry, 172*, 308–313.

Malzberg, B. (1967). Internal migration and mental disease among the white population of New York state, 1960–1961. *International Journal of Social Psychiatry, 13*, 184–191.

Marcelis, M., Navarro-Mateu, F., Murray, R., Selten, J.P., & van Os, J. (1998). Urbanization and psychosis: a study of 1942–1978 birth cohorts in the Netherlands. *Psychological Medicine, 28*, 871–879.

Margari, F., Presicci, A., Petruzzelli, M.G., Ventura, P., Di Cuonzo, F., & Palma, M., et al. (2008). Very early onset and greater vulnerability in schizophrenia: A clinical and neuroimaging study. *Neuropsychiatric Disease and Treatment, 4*, 825–830.

Mata, I., Beperet, M., Madoz, V., & Psicost, Y. (2000). Prevalence and incidence of schizophrenia in Navarra. *Anales Sis San Navara, 23*, 29–36.

Matson, J.L., & Boisjoli, J.A. (2009). The token economy for children with intellectual disability and/or autism: A review. *Research in Developmental Disabilities, 30*, 240–248.

Matsumoto, H., Simmons, A., Williams, S., Pipe, R., Murray, R., & Frangou, S. (2001). Structural magnetic imaging of the hippocampus in early onset schizophrenia. *Biological Psychiatry, 49*, 824–831.

Maurer, K., & Hafner, H. (1995). Methodological aspects of onset assessment in schizophrenia. *Schizophrenia Research, 15*, 265–276.

Maziade, M., Bouchard, S., Gingras, N., Charron, L., Cardinal, A., Roy, M.A., & Martinez, M. (1996). Long-term stability of diagnosis and symptom dimensions in a systematic sample of patients with onset of schizophrenia in childhood and early adolescence. II: positive/negative distinction and childhood predictors of adult outcome. *British Journal of Psychiatry, 169*, 371–378.

McClellan, J.M., Breiger, D., McCurry, C., & Hlastala, S.A. (2003). Premorbid functioning in early onset psychotic disorders. *Journal of the American Academy of Child and Adolescent Psychiatry, 42*(6), 666–672.

McClellan, J., & Werry, J. (2001). Practice parameters for the assessment and treatment of children and adolescents with schizophrenia. *Journal of the American Academy of Child and Adolescent Psychiatry, 40*(S), 4S–23S.

McFarlane, W.R., Lukens, E., Link, B., Dushay, R., Deakins, S.A., Newmark, M., & Toran, J. (1995). Multiple-family groups and psychoeducation in the treatment of schizophrenia. *Archives of General Psychiatry, 52*, 679–687.

McGorry, P.D., McFarlane, C., Patton, G.C., Bell, R., Hibbert, M.E., Jackson, H.J., & Bowes, G. (1995). The prevalence of prodromal features of schizophrenia in adolescence: A preliminary survey. *Acta Psychiatrica Scandinavica, 92*, 241–249.

McGovern, D. & Cope, R.V. (1987). First psychiatric admission rates of first and second generation Afro-Caribbeans. *Social Psychiatry, 22*,139–149.

McGrath, J. (1999). Hypothesis: Is low prenatal vitamin D a risk modifying factor for schizophrenia? *Schizophrenia Research, 40*, 173–177.

McNaught, A.S., Jeffreys, S.E., Harvey, C.A., Quayle, A.S., King, M.B., & Bird, A.S. (1997). The Hampstead Schizophrenia Survey 1991. II: Incidence and migration in inner London. *British Journal of Psychiatry, 170*, 307–311.

McNeil, T.F. (1988). Obstetric factors and perinatal injuries. In M.T. Tsuang, D.C. Simpson, (eds), *Handbook of schizophrenia Vol. 3: Nosology, epidemiology and genetics* (pp. 319–343). New York, NY: Elsvier Science Publication Co.

Meadows, G., Turner, T., Campbell, L., Lewis, S.W., Reveley, M.A. & Murray, R.M. (1991). Assessing schizophrenia in adults with mental retardation: a comparative study. *British Journal of Psychiatry, 158*, 103–105.

Mehler, C., & Warnke, A. (2002). Structural brain abnormalities specific to childhood-onset schizophrenia identified by neuroimaging techniques. *Journal of Neural Transmission, 109*, 219–234.

Messias, E., Sampaio, J.J., Messias, N.C., & Kirkpatrick, B. (2000). Epidemiology of schizophrenia in Northeast Brazil. *Journal of Nervous and Mental Disorders, 188*, 118–120.

Meyer, U., & Feldon, J. (2009). Prenatal exposure to infection: a primary mechanism for abnormal dopaminergic development in schizophrenia. *Psychopharmacology, 206*, 587–602.
Mezey, A.G., & Evans, E. (1971). Psychiatric in-patients and out-patients in a London borough. *British Journal of Psychiatry, 118*, 609–616.
Miller, T.J., Cicchetti, D., Markovich, P.J., McGlashan, T.H. & Woods, S.W. (2004). The SIPS screen: A brief self-report screen to detect the schizophrenia prodrome. *Schizophrenia Research*, 70(supp.), 78.
Miller, R., & Mason, S. (2002). *Diagnosis: Schizophrenia*. New York: Columbia University Press.
Miller, T.J., McGlashan, T.H., Rosen, J.L., Cadenhead, K., Ventura, J., McFarlane, W., & Woods, S.W. (2003). Prodromal assessment with the Structure Interview for Prodromal Symptoms: Predictive validity, interrater reliability, and training to reliability. *Schizophrenia Bulletin, 29*, 703–715.
Morgan, C., & Fisher, H. (2007). Environmental factors in schizophrenia: Childhood trauma–A critical review. *Schizophrenia Bulletin, 33*, 3–10.
Morgan, V.A., Leonard, H., & Jablensky, A. (2008). Intellectual disability co-occurring with schizophrenia and other psychiatric illness: population-based study. *The British Journal of Psychiatry, 193*, 364–372.
Morrison, A. (2001). The interpretation of intrusions in psychosis: an integrative cognitive approach to hallucinations and delusions. *Behavioral cognitive Therapy, 29*, 257–276.
Mors, O., & Sorensen, L.V. (1993). Incidence and comorbidity of psychiatric disorders from a well-defined catchment area in Denmark. *European Psychiatry, 8*, 193–199.
Mortensen, P.B., Pederson, C.B., Westergaard, T., Wohlfahrt, J., Ewald, H., Mors, O., & Mads (1999). Effects of family history and place and season of birth on the risk of schizophrenia. *New England Journal of Medicine, 340*, 603–608.
Mowry, B.J., & Nancarrow, D.J. (2001). Molecular genetics of schizophrenia. *Clinical and Experimental Pharmacology and Physiology, 28*, 66–69.
Mozes, T., Greenberg, Y., Spivak, B., Tyano, S., Weizman, A., & Mester, R. (2003). Olanzapine treatment in chronic-drug resistant childhood-onset schizophrenia: An open-label study. *Journal of Child and Adolescent Psychopharmacology, 13*, 311–317.
Mueser, K., & Bond, G.R. (2000). Psychosocial treatment approaches for schizophrenia. *Current Opinion in Psychiatry, 13*, 27–35.
Mueser, K.T., & McGurk, S.R. (2004). Schizophrenia. *The Lancet, 363*, 2063–72.
Mullins, D., Pfefferbaum B., Schultz, H., & Overall, J.E. (1986). Brief psychiatric rating scale for children: Quantitative scoring of medical records. *Psychiatry Research, 19*, 43–49.
Munk-Jorgensen, P. (1986). Decreasing first-admission rates of schizophrenia among males in Denmark from 1970 to 1984. Changing diagnostic patterns? *Acta Psychiatrica Scandinavica, 73*, 645–650.
Munk-Jorgensen, P., Lutzhoft, J.H., Jensen, J., & Stromgren, E. (1992). Trends in psychiatric hospitalization in Denmark: A10-year register-based investigation. *Acta Psychiatrica Scandinavica, 86*, 79–83.
Munk-Jorgensen P. & Mortensen, P.B. (1992). Social outcome in schizophrenia: A 13-year follow-up. *Social Psychiatry and Psychiatric Epidemiology, 27*(3), 129–134.
Munk-Jorgensen, P., & Mortensen, P.B. (1992) Incidence and other aspects of the epidemiology of schizophrenia in Denmark, 1971–87. *British Journal of Psychiatry, 161*, 489–495.
Muratori, F., Salvadori, F., D'Arcangelo, G., Viglione, V., & Picchi, L. (2005). Childhood psychopathological antecedents in early onset schizophrenia. *European psychiatry, 20*, 309–14.
Myles-Worsley, M., Blailes, F., Ord, L.M., Weaver, S., Dever, G., & Faraone, S.V. (2007). The Palau Early Psychosis Study: Distribution of cases by level of genetic risk. *American Journal of Medical Genetics Part B: Neuropsychiatric Genetics, 144B*, 5–9.
Neehall, J. (1991). An analysis of psychiatric inpatient admissions from a defined geographic catchment area over a one-year period. *West Indian Medicine Journal, 40*, 16–21.
Niendam, T.A., Bearden, C.E., Johnson, J.K., McKinley, M., Loewy, R., O'Brien, M., Cannon, T.D. (2006). Neurocognitive performance and functional disability in the psychosis prodrome. *Schizophrenia Research, 84*, 100–111.

Ni Nuallain, M., O'Hare, A., Walsh, D., Blake, B., Halpenny, J.N., & O'Brien, P.F. (1984). The incidence of mental illness in Ireland–patients contacting psychiatric services in three Irish counties. *Irish Journal of Psychiatry, 5*, 23–29.

Nicolson, R., Brookner, F. B., Lenane Gochman, P., Ingraham, L.J., Egan, M.F., & Rapoport, J.L. (2003). Parental schizophrenia spectrum disorders in childhood-onset and adult on-set schizophrenia. *American Journal of Psychiatry, 160*, 490–495.

Nicole, L., Lesage, A., & Lalonde, P. (1992). Lower incidence and increased male: female ratio in schizophrenia. *British Journal of Psychiatry, 161*, 556–557.

Nicolson, R., Lenane, M., Hamburger, S.D., Fernandez, T., Bedwell, J., & Rapoport, J. L. (2000). Lessons from childhood-onset schizophrenia. *Brain Research Reviews, 31*, 147–156.

Nicolson, R., & Rapoport, J.L. (1999). Childhood-onset schizophrenia: Rare but worth studying. *Biological Psychiatry, 46*, 1418–1428.

Nielsen, J. (1976). The Samso project from 1957 to 1974. *Acta Psychiatrica Scandinavica, 54*, 198–222.

Nielsen, J., & Nielsen, J.A. (1977). A census study of mental illness in Samso. *Psychological Medicine, 7*, 491–503.

Niskanen, P., & Achte, K.A. (1972). The course and prognosis of schizophrenic psychoses in helsinki, a comparative study of first admissions in 1960 and 1965. Helsinki; Helsinki University Central Hospital.

Odegar, O. (1932). Emigration and insanity: A study of mental disease among Norwegian born population in Minnesota. *Acta Psychiatrica Neurologica Scandinavica, 4*.

O'Hare, A., & Walsh, D. (1974). Further data on activities of Irish psychiatric hospitals and units, 1965–1969. *Journal of Irish Medicine Association, 67*, 57–63.

Ohta, Y., Nakane, Y., Nishihara, J., & Takemoto, T. (1992). Ecological structure and incidence rates of schizophrenia in Nagasaki City. *Acta Psychiatrica Scandinavica, 86*, 113–120.

Oldehinkel, A.J., & Giel, R. (1995). Time trends in the care-based incidence of schizophrenia. *British Journal of Psychiatry, 167*, 777–782.

Olsen, K.A., & Rosenbaum, B. (2006). Prospective investigations of the prodromal state of schizophrenia: Assessment instruments. *Acta Psychiatrica Scandinavica, 113*, 273–282.

O'Neill, R.E., Horner, R.H., Albin, R.W., Sprague, J.R., Storey, K. & Newton, J.S. (1997). *Functional Assessment and Program Development for Problem Behavior: A Practical Handbook* (2nd ed.). Pacific Grove, CA: Brooks/Cole.

Opler, M.G.A., Buka, S.L., Groeger, J., McKeague, I., Wei, C., Factor-Litvak, P., & Susser, E.S. (2008). Prenatal exposure to lead, alpha aminolevulinic acid, and schizophrenia: Further evidence. *Environmental Health Perspectives, 116*, 1586–1590.

Opler, M.G.A., & Susser, E.S. (2005). Fetal environment and schizophrenia. *Environmental Health Perspectives, 113*, 1239–1242.

Ord, L.M., Myles-Worsley, M., Blailes, F., & Ngiralmau, H. (2004). Screening for prodromal adolescents in an isolated high risk population. *Schizophrenia Research, 71*, 507–508.

Orr, K., & Castle, D.J. (2003). Schizophrenia at the extremes of life. In: R. Murray, P.B. Jones, E. Susser, J. van Os, & M. Cannon (Eds.), *The Epidemiology of Schizophrenia* (pp.167–184). Cambridge, MA: University Press.

Ösby, U., Hammar, N., Brandt, L., Wicks, S., Thinsz, Z., Ekbom, A., & Sparén, P. (2001). Time trends in first admissions for schizophrenia and paranoid psychosis in Stockholm County, Sweden. *Schizophrenia Research, 47*, 247–254.

Parnas, J., Handest, P., Saebye, D., & Jansson, L. (2003). Anomalies of subjective experience in schizophrenia and psychotic bipolar illness. *Acta Psychiatrica Scandinavica, 108*, 126–133.

Patel, N. C., Crismon, M.L., Shafer, A., De Leon, A., Lopez, M., & Lane, D.C. (2006). Ethnic variation in symptoms and responses to risperidone in youth with schizophrenia-spectrum disorders. *Social Psychiatry and Psychiatric Epidemiology, 41*, 341–346.

Patterson, Ph. H. (2007). Maternal effects on schizophrenia risk. *Science, 318*, 576–577.

Paul, G.L., & Lentz, R.J. (1977). *Psychosocial treatment of chronic mental patients: milieu versus social learning programs*. Cambridge, Mass, Harvard University Press.

Peen, J., & Dekker, J. (1997). Admission rates for schizophrenia in The Netherlands: Anurban/rural comparison. *Acta Psychiatrica Scandinavica, 96*, 301–305.

Penn, D.L., Mueser, K.T., Tarrier, N., Gloege, A., Cather, C., Serrano, D., & Otto, M.W. (2004). Supportive therapies for schizophrenia: Possible mechanisms and implications for adjunctive psychosocial treatments. *Schizophrenia Bulletin, 30*, 101–112.

Phillips, T.J., James, A.C.D., Crow, T.J., & Collinson, S.L. (2004). Semantic fluency in impaired but phonemic and design fluency are preserved in early-onset schizophrenia. *Schizophrenia Research, 70*, 215–222.

Phillips, L.J., McGorry, P.D., Yung, A.R., McGlashan, T.H., Cornblatt, B., & Klosterkotter, J. (2005). Prepsychotic phase of schizophrenia and related disorders: Recent progress and future opportunities. *British Journal of Psychiatry, 187* (suppl. 48), s33–s44.

Pilling, S., Bebbington, P., Kuipers, E., Garety, P., Geddes, J., Orbach, G., & Morgan, C. (2002). Psychological treatments in schizophrenia: II. Meta-analyses of randomized controlled trials of social skills training and cognitive remediation. *Psychological Medicine, 32*, 783–791.

Pinto, A., La Pia, S., Mennella, R., Giorgio, D., & DeSimone, L. (1999). Cognitive behavioral therapy and clozapine for clients with treatment-refractory schizophrenia. *Psychiatric Services, 50*, 901–904.

Pitschel-Walz, G., Leucht, S., Bauml, J., Kissling, W., & Engel, R.R. (2001). The effect of family interventions on relapse and rehospitalization in schizophrenia –a meta-analysis. *Schizophrenia Bulletin, 27*, 73–92.

Potash, J. B., Willour, V. L., Chiu, Y. F., Simpson, S. G., MacKinnon, D. F., & McInnis, M.G. (2001). The familial aggregation of psychotic symptoms in bipolar disorder pedigrees. *American Journal of Psychiatry, 158*, 1258–1264.

Poulton, R., Caspi, A., Moffitt, T. E., Cannon, M., Murray, R., & Harrington, H. (2000). Children's self-reported psychotic symptoms and adult schizophreniform disorder: A 15-year longitudinal study. *Archives of General Psychiatry, 57*, 1053–1058.

Preti, A., & Miotto, P. (2000). Increase in first admissions for schizophrenia and other major psychoses in Italy. *Psychiatry Research, 94*, 139–152.

Prince, M., & Phelan, M. (1990). Trends in Schizophrenia. *Lancet, 335*, 851–852.

Prince, M., & Phelan, M. (1994). Invisible schizophrenia: A postal survey of the incidence and management of new cases of schizophrenia in primary care. *Journal of Mental Health, 3*, 91–98.

Rajkumar, S., Padmavati, R., Thara, R., & Sarada Menon, M. (1993). Incidence of schizophrenia in an urban community in Madras. *Indian Journal of Psychiatry, 35*, 18–21.

Raman, A.C. & Murphy, H.B. (1972). Failure of traditional prognostic indications in Afro-Asian psychotics: results of a long-term follow-up survey. *The Journal of nervous and mental disease, 154*(4), 238–247.

Rasanan, P., Tiihonen, J., Isohanni, M., Rantakillio, P., Lehtonen, J. & Moring, T. (1998). Schizophrenia alcohol abuse and violent behaviour: A 26 year followup study of an unselected birth cohort. *Schizophrenia Bulletin, 24*, 437–441.

Reichert, A., Kreiker, S., Mehler-Wex, C., & Warnke, A. (2008). The psychopathological and psychosocial outcome of early-onset schizophrenia: Preliminary data of a 13-year follow-up. *Child and Adolescent Psychiatry and Mental Health, 2*, 6.

Read J, van Os J, Morrison A.P., & Ross C.A. (2005). Childhood trauma, psychosis and schizophrenia: A literature review with theoretical and clinical implications. *Acta Psychiatry Scandinavia*, 112, 330–350.

Reaven, J.A., Hepburn, S.L., & Randal, G. (2008). Use of the ADS and ADI-R in children with psychosis: Importance of clinical judgment. *Clinical Child Psychology and Psychiatry, 13*, 81–94.

Reid, A. (1989). Schizophrenia in mental retardation: Clinical features. *Research in Developmental Disabilities, 10* (3), 241–249.

Remschmidt, H. (2002). Early-onset schizophrenia as a progressive-deteriorating developmental disorder: Evidence from child psychiatry. *Journal of Neural Transmission, 109*, 101–117.

Remschmidt, H., & Theisen, F.M. (2005). Schizophrenia and related disorders in children and adolescents. *Journal of Neural Transmission, 69*, 121–141.

Repetto, F., Formigaro, F., Ferrari, P., Frascaroli, G., Lora, A., Magnani, G., Morosini, P. (1988). Estimate of the hospital incidence of schizophrenia in Lombardy. *Epidemiologia E Prevenzione, 10*, 20–25.

Reynolds, C. R., & Kamphaus, R.W. (2004). *Behavior Assessment System for Children* (2nd edition). Pearson, Inc.

Rhinewine, J.P., Lencz, T., Thaden, E.P., Cervellione, K.L., Burdick, K.E., Henderson, I., Bhaskar, S, Kumra, S. (2005). Neurocognitive profile in adolescents with early-onset schizophrenia: Clinical correlates. *Biological Psychiatry, 58*, 705–712.

Riecher, A., Maurer, K., Loffler, W., Fatkenheuer, B., van der Heiden, W., Munk-Jorgenson, P. et al. (1990). Gender differences in age at onset and course of schizophrenic disorders. In H. Hafner and W. F. Gattaz (eds.), *Search for the Causes of Schizophrenia* (pp. 14–33). Berlin Heidelberg: Springer-Verlag.

Riecher-Rossler, A., Gschwandtner, U., Borgwardt, S., Aston, J., Pfluger, M., & Rossler, W. (2006). Early detection and treatment of schizophrenia: How early? *Acta Psychiatrica Scandinavica, 113* (Suppl 429), 73–80.

Ring, N., Tantam, D., Montague, L., Newby, D., Black, D., & Morris, J. (1991). Gender differences in the incidence of definite schizophrenia and atypical psychosis –focus on negative symptoms of schizophrenia. *Acta Psychiatrica Scandinavica, 84*, 489–496.

Robins, L. (1996). *Deviant children growing up*. London: Williams Wilkins.

Ross, R.G., Novins, D., Farley, G.K., & Adler, L.E. (2003). A 1-Year open-label trial of olanzapine in school-age children with schizophrenia. *Journal of Child and Adolescent Psychopharmacology, 13*, 301–309.

Ross, R.G., Schaeffer, J., Compagnon, N., Heinlen, S., Beresford, C., & Farley, G. (2003). Creating school-age versions of semistructured interviews for the prodrome to schizophrenia: Lessons from case reviews. *Schizophrenia Bulletin, 29*, 729–735.

Rotshtein, V.G. (1982). Incidence of paranoid schizophrenia. *Zhurnal nevropatologii i psikhiatrii imeni S.S. Korsakova, 82*, 91–98.

Rowland, A. S., Lesesne, C.A., & Abramowitz, A.J. (2002). The epidemiology of attention-deficit/hyperactivity disorder (ADHD): A public health view. *Mental Retardation and Developmental Disabilities Research Reviews, 8*, 162–170.

Russell, A.T., Bott, L., & Sammons, C. (1989). The phenomenology of schizophrenia occurring in childhood. *Journal of the American Academy of Child and Adolescent Psychiatry, 28*, 399–407.

Rwegellera, G.G. (1977). Psychiatric morbidity among West Africans and West Indians living in London. *Psychological Medicine, 7*, 317–329.

Schaeffer, J.L., & Ross, R.G. (2002). Childhood-onset schizophrenia: Premorbid and prodromal diagnostic and treatment histories. *Journal of American Academy of Child and Adolescent Psychiatry, 41*, 538–545.

Schioiri, T., Shinada, K., Kuwabara, H., & Someya, T. (2007). Early prodromal symptoms and diagnoses before first psychotic episode in 219 inpatients with schizophrenia. *Psychiatry and Clinical Neuroscience, 61*, 348–354.

Schultze-Lutter, F., Ruhrmann, S., Picker, H., & Klosterkotter, J. (2006). The schizophrenia proneness instrument (SPI-A)—a tool for the assessment of basic symptoms. *European Psychiatry*, 21 (suppl. 1), s27.

Schultze-Lutter, F., Ruhrmann, S., Picker, H., & von Reventlow, H.G. (2007). Basic symptoms in early psychotic and depressive disorders. *British Journal of Psychiatry, 191*, s31–s37.

Seidman, L.J., Giuliano, A.J., Smith, C.W., Stone, W.S., Glatt, S.J., Meyer, E., Cornblatt, B. (2006). Neuropsychological functioning in adolescents and young adults at genetic risk for schizophrenia and affective psychosis: Results from the Harvard and Hillside adolescent high risk studies. *Schizophrenia Bulletin, 32*, 507–524.

Seiferth, N.Y., Pauly, K., Kellermann, T., Shah, N.J., Ott, G., Herpertz-Dahlmann, B., Habel, U. (2009). Neuronal correlates of facial emotion discrimination in early onset schizophrenia. *Neuropsychopharmacology, 34*, 477–487.

Shaffer, D., Fisher, P., Lucas, C.P., Dulcan, M.K., & Schwab-Stone, M.E. (2000). NIMH Diagnostic Interview Schedule for Children Version IV (NIMH DISC-IV): description, differences from

previous versions, and reliability of some common diagnoses. *Journal of American Academy Child Adolescence Psychiatry, 39*, 28–38.
Shaffer, D., Gould, M.S., Brasic, J., Ambrosini, P., Fisher, P., & Bird, H., & Aluwahlia, S. (1983). A children's global assessment scale(CGAS). *Archives of General Psychiatry, 40*, 1228–1231.
Shen, W.W. (1999). A history of antipsychotic drug development. *Comprehensive Psychiatry, 40*, 407–414.
Shin, L., Bregman, H., Frazier, J., & Noyes, N. (2008). An overview of obesity in children with psychiatric disorders taking atypical antipsychotics. *Harvard Review of Psychiatry, 16*, 69–79.
Sikich, L. (2005). Individual psychotherapy and school interventions for psychotic youth. In R.L. Findling & S.C. Schulz (Eds.), *Juvenile-Onset Schizophrenia: Assessment, Neurobiology, and Treatment*. (pp. 257–287).Baltimore, MD: John Hopkins Press.
Sikich, L., Frazier, J.A., McClellan, J., Findling, R.L., Vitiello, B., Ritz, L., & Lieberman, J.A. (2008). Double-blind comparison of first- and second-generation antipsychotics in early-onset schizophrenia and schizoaffective disorder: Findings from the Treatment of Early-Onset Schizophrenia Spectrum Disorders (TEOSS) study. *American Journal of Psychiatry, 165*, 1420–1431.
Simon, A.E., Dvorsky, D.N., Boesch, J., Roth, B., Isler, E., Schueler, P., & Umbricht, D. (2006). Defining subjects at risk for psychosis: A comparison of two approaches. *Schizophrenia Research, 81*, 83–90.
Smith, P. (2007). Have we made any progress? Including students with intellectual disabilities in regular education classrooms. *Intellectual and Developmental Disabilities, 45*, 297–309.
Soleil, G. (2000). *AD/HD and school law*. Washington, DC: Office of Educational Research and Improvement. Retrieved November 5, 2006 from www.eric.ed.gov/sitemap/html_0900000b8013425b.html
Sorensen, H.J., Mortensen, E.L., Parnas, J., & Mednick, S.A. (2006). Premorbid neurocognitive functioning in schizophrenia spectrum disorders. *Schizophrenia Bulletin, 32*, 578–583.
Sørensen, H. J., Mortensen, E. L., Reinisch, J. M., & Mednick, S. (2003). Do hypertension and diuretic treatment in pregnancy increase the risk of schizophrenia in offspring? *American Journal of Psychiatry, 160*, 464–468.
Sowell, E. R., Levitt, J., Thompson, P. M., Holmes, C. J., Blanton, R. E., Kornsand, D.S., & Toga, A.W. (2000). Brain abnormalities in early-onset schizophrenia spectrum disorder observed with statistical parametric mapping of structural magnetic resonance images. *American Journal of Psychiatry, 157*, 1475—1484.
Sparrow, S.S., Balla, D.A., & Cichetti, D.V. (1984). *Vineland Adaptive Behavior Scales*. Circle Pines, MH: American Guidance Services.
Stefansson, H., Rujescu, D., Cichon, S., Pietiläinen, O. P. H., Ingason, A., & Steinberg, S. (2008). Large recurrent microdeletions associated with schizophrenia. *Nature, 455*, 232–236.
Susser, E. S., Neugebauer, R., Hoek H. W., Brown, A. S., Lin, S., Labovitzet, D., & Gorman, J.M. (1996). Schizophrenia after prenatal famine: Further evidence. *Archives of General Psychiatry, 53*, 25–31.
Tandon, R., Nasrallah, H. A., & Keshavan, M. S. (2009). Schizophrenia, "just the facts" 4. Clinical features and conceptualization. *Schizophrenia Research, 110*, 1–23.
Tansella, M., Balestrieri, M., Meneghelli, M., & Micciolo, R.l. (1991). Trends in the provision of psychiatric care 1979–1988. *Psychological Medicine 19*, 1–54.
Taub, J. & Pearrow, M. (2007). School functioning for children enrolled in community based wrap-around services. In C. Newman, C.J. Liberton, K. Kutash & R. Friedman, (Eds.), *The 19th Annual Research Conference Proceedings: A System of Care for Children's Mental Health: Expanding the Research Base* (pp. 323–326). Tampa: University of South Florida, Louis de la Parte Florida Mental Health Institute, Research and Training Center for Children's Mental Health.
Taylor, M., Carlson, S.M., Maring, B.L., Gerow, L., & Charley, C.M. (2004). The characteristics and correlates of fantasy in school-age children: Imaginary companions, impersonation, and social understanding. *Developmental Psychology, 40*, 1173–1187.
Taylor, P.J., & Gunn, J. (1984). Violence and psychosis. I. Risk of violence among psychotic men. *British Medical Journal, 288*, 1945–1949.

The Psychological Corporation. (2002). *Wechsler Individual Achievement Tests –Second Edition.* San Antonio, TX: Author.

Thomas, C.S., Stone, K., Osborn, M., Thomas, P.F., & Fisher, M. (1993). Psychiatric morbidity and compulsory admission among UK-born Europeans, Afro-Caribbeans and Asians in central Manchester. *British Journal of Psychiatry, 163*, 91–99.

Thomsen, P. (1996). Schizophrenia with childhood and adolescent onset- a nationwide register-based study. *Acta Psychiatrica Scandinavica, 94*, 187–193.

Tien, A.Y., & Eaton, W.W. (1992). Psychopathologic precursors and sociodemographic risk factors for the schizophrenia syndrome. *Archives of General Psychiatry, 49*, 37–46.

Tienari, P., Wynne, L. C., Moring, J., Lahti, I., Naarala, M., Sorri A., et al. (1994). The Finnish adoptive family study of schizophrenia: Implications for family research. *British Journal of Psychiatry, 23*, supplement, 27–28.

Tomoras, V., Mavreas, V., Economou, M., Ioannovich, E., Karydi, V., & Siefanis, C. (2000). The effect of family intervention on chronic schizophrenics under individual psychosocial treatment: A 3-year study. *Social Psychiatry and Psychiatric Epidemiology, 35*, 487–493.

Torrey, E.F., Miller, J., Rawlings, R., & Yolken, R. H. (1997). Seasonality of births in schizophrenia and bipolar disorder: A review of the literature. *Schizophrenia Research*, 28, 1–38.

Tsoi, W.F., & Chen, A.J. (1979). New admissions to Woodbridge Hospital 1975 with special reference to schizophrenia. *Academy of Medicine Singapore, 8*, 275–279.

Tsuang, M.T., Stone, W. S., & Faraone, S. V. (2001). Genes, environment and schizophrenia. *British Journal of Psychiatry*, 40S: 18–24.

Turner, T.H. (1989). Schizophrenia and mental handicap: A historical review with implications for further research. *Psychological medicine, 19*, 301–314.

Tuulio-Henriksson, A., Partonen, T., Suvisaari, J., Haukka, J., & Lonnqvist, J. (2004). Age at onset and cognitive functioning in schizophrenia. *British Journal of Psychiatry, 185*, 215–219.

Tyrer S.P., & Dunstan J.A. (1997) Schizophrenia. In S. G. Read (Ed), *Psychiatry in Learning Disability* (185–215), London: W.B. Saunders Company Ltd.

U.S. Department of Health and Human Services (1999). *Mental Health: A Report of the Surgeon General.* Rockville, MD: U.S. Department of Health and Human Services, Substance Abuse and Mental Health Services Administration, Center for Mental Health Services, National Institutes of Health, National Institute of Mental Health.

U.S. Department of Health and Human Services. (n.d.). Evidence-based practices: Shaping mental health services toward recovery: Assertive community treatment. Retrieved June 9, 2007 from http://mentalhealth.samhsa.gov/cmhs/communitysupport/toolkits/community/ACTinfoPMHA.asp

van Os, J., Castle, D.J., Takei, N., Der, G., & Murray, R.M. (1996). Psychotic illness in ethnic minorities: clarification from the 1991 census. *Psychological Medicine, 26*, 203–208.

van Os, J., Driessen, G., Gunther, N., & Delespaul, P. (2000). Neighbourhood variation in incidence of schizophrenia. Evidence for person-environment interaction. *British Journal of Psychiatry, 176*, 243–248.

van Os, J., Galdos, P., Lewis, G., Bourgeois, M., & Mann, A. (1993). Schizophrenia sans frontieres: Concepts of schizophrenia among French and British psychiatrists. *British Medical Journal, 307*, 489–492.

Van Zelst, C. (2009). Stigmatization as an environmental risk in schizophrenia: A user perspective. *Schizophrenia Bulletin, 35*, 293–296.

Vazquez-Barquero, J.L., Cuesta Nunez, M.J., de la Varga, M., Herrera Castanedo, S., Gaite, L., & Arenal, A. (1995). The Cantabria first episode schizophrenia study: a summary of general findings. *Acta Psychiatrica Scandinavica, 91*, 156–162.

Verdoux, H., Geddes, J. R., Takei, N., Lawrie, S. M., Bover, P., Murray, R.M. (1997). Obstetric complications and age at onset in schizophrenia: An international collaborative meta-analysis of individual patient data. *American Journal of Psychiatry, 154*, 1220–1227.

Vidal, C.N., Rapoport, J.L., Hayashi, K. M., Geaga, J.A., Sui, Y., McLemore, L.E., Thompson, P.M. (2006). Dynamically spreading frontal and cingulate deficits mapped in adolescents with schizophrenia. *Archives of General psychiatry, 63*, 25–34.

Volavka, J., Laska, E., Baker, S., Meisner, M., Czobor, P., & Krivelevich, I. (1997). History of violent behaviour and schizophrenia in different cultures. Analyses based on the WHO study on determinants of outcome of severe mental disorders. *British Journal of Psychiatry, 171*: 9–14.

Volkmar, F.R., & Cohen, D.J. (1991). Comorbid association of autism and schizophrenia. *The American Journal of Psychiatry, 148* (12), 1705–1707.

Vollmer-Larsen, A., Handest, P., & Parnas, J. (2007). Reliability of measuring anomalous experience: The Bonn Scale for the Assessment of Basic Symptoms. *Psychopathology, 40*, 345–348.

Vourdas, A., Pipe, R., Corrigall, R., & Frangou, S. (2003). Increased developmental deviance and premorbid dysfunction in early onset schizophrenia. *Schizophrenia Research*, 62–1 3–22.

Vul, F.R., Mishkind, A.D., Gil'burd, O.A., & Vorobeichik, D.A. (1988). Clinico-epidemiologic characteristics of mental diseases in one of the regions of western Siberia. *Zhurnal nevropatologii i psikhiatrii imeni S.S. Korsakova, 88*, 111–116.

Walder, D.J., Seidman, L.J., Cullen, N., Su, J., Tsuang, M.T., & Goldstein, J.M. (2006). Sex differences in language dysfunction in schizophrenia. American Journal of Psychiatry, *163*, 470–477.

Walker, E.F. (2002). Adolescent neurodevelopment and psychopathology. *Current Directions in Psychological Science, 11*, 24–28.

Walker, J.S. (2008). How, and why, does wraparound work: A theory of change. In E. J. Bruns & J.S. Walker (Eds.), *The resource guide to wraparound*. Portland, OR: National Wraparound Initiative, Research and Training Center for Family Support and Children's Mental Health.

Walker E., & Diforio, D. (1997). Schizophrenia: A neural diathesis-stress model. *Psychological Review, 104*, 67–685.

Walker, E., Kestler, L., Bollini, A., & Hochman, K. (2004). Schizophrenia: Etiology and course. *Annual Review of Psychology. 55*: 401–430.

Walker, E.F., Kestler, L.P., Hochman, K.M., & Bollini, A.M. (2005). Development during childhood and adolescence: The manifestations of impending schizophrenia. In R.L. Findling & S.C. Schulz (Eds.), *Juvenile Onset Schizophrenia: Assessment, Neurobiology, and Treatment.* (pp. 174–198). Baltimore, MD: The John Hopkins University Press.

Walker, E., & Lewine, R. (1990). Prediction of adult-onset schizophrenia from childhood home movies of the patients. *American Journal of Psychiatry, 147*, 1052–1056.

Walker, Z., & Seifer, R. (1994). Violent incidents in a psychiatric intensive care unit. *British Journal of Psychiatry, 164*, 826–828.

Wallace, C., Mullen, P., Burgess, P., Palmer, S., Ruschena, D., & Browne, C. (1998). Serious criminal offending and mental disorder. Case linkage study. *British Journal of Psychiatry, 174*, 477–484.

Walsh, D. (1969). Mental illness in Dublin –first admissions. *British Journal Psychiatry, 115*, 449–456.

Walsh, D. (1992). The ups and downs of schizophrenia in Ireland. *Irish Journal Psychiatry, 13*, 12–16.

Walsh, E., & Buchana, A. (2006). Criminal and violent behaviour in schizohrenia. In: R.M. Murray, P. Jones, E. Susser, J. van Os, & M. Cannon (Eds.), *The Epidemiology of Schizophrenia* (pp. 343–357). Cambridge, MA: University Press.

Watson, A.C., Otey, E., Westbrook, A.L., Gardner, A.L., Lamb, T.A., Corrigan, P.W., & Fenton, W.S. (2004). Changing middle schoolers' attitudes about mental illness through education. *Schizophrenia Bulletin, 30*, 563–572.

Wechsler, D. (2003). *Wechsler Intelligence Scale for Children* (4th edition). (WISC-IV). San Antonio, TX: Psychological Corporation.

Wechsler, D. (2009). *Wechsler Individual Achievement Test* (3rd ed.). (WIAT-III). Bloomington, MN: Pearson.

Welham, J., Isohanni, M., Jones, P., & McGrath, (2009). The antecedents of schizophrenia: A review of birth cohort studies. *Schizophrenia Bulletin, 35*, 603–623.

Werry, J.S., McClellan, J.M., & Chard, L. (1991). Childhood and adolescent schizophrenic, bipolar, and schizoaffective disorders: a clinical and outcome study. *Journal of the American Academy of Child and Adolescent Psychiatry, 30*, 457–465.

Weyerer, S., & Hafner, H. (1992). The high incidence of psychiatrically treated disorders in the inner city of Mannheim. Susceptibility of German and foreign residents. *Social Psychiatry and Psychiatric Epidemiology, 27*, 142–146.

Wiersma, D., Nienhuis, F.J., & Stooff, C.J. (1998). Natural course of schizophrenia disorders: A 15-year follow-up of a Dutch incidence cohort. *Schizophrenia Bulletin, 24*, 75–85.

Wilens, T.E. (2009). *Straight talk about psychiatric medications for kids* (3rd ed.). New York: Guilford Press.

Willinger, U., Heiden, A. M., Meszaros, K., Formann, A.K., & Aschauer, H. N. (2001). Neurodevelopmental schizophrenia: Obstetric complications, birth weight, premorbid social withdrawal and learning disabilities. *Neuropsychobiology, 43* (3), 163–169.

Wolwer, W., Buchkremer, G., Hafner, H., Klosterkotter, J., Maier, W., Moller, J, & Gaebel, W. (2003). German research network on schizophrenia: Bridging the gap between research and care. *European Archive of Psychiatry Clinical Neuroscience, 253*, 321–329.

Woodberry, K.A., Giuliano, A.J., & Seidman, L.J. (2008). Premorbid IQ in schizophrenia: A meta-analytic review. *The American Journal of Psychiatry, 165*, 579–587.

Woodcock, R., McGrew, K., & Mather, N. (2001). *Woodcock Johnson III Tests of Achievement*. Itasca, IL: Riverside Publishing.

Woods, S. W., Miller, T. J., & McGlashan, T. H. (2001b). The prodromal patient: Both symptomatic and at risk. *CNS Spectrums, 6*, 223–232.

Wood, S. J., Pantelis, C., Proffitt, T., Phillips, L. J., Stuart, G. W., Buchanan, J., Mahony, K., Brewer, W.J., Smith, D., & McGorry, P.D. (2003). Spatial working memory ability is a marker of risk-for-psychosis. *Psychological Medicine 33*:1239–1247.

Worthington, J., Hernandez, M., Friedman, B., & Uzzell, D. (2001). *Systems of Care: Promising Practices in Children's Mental Health, 2001 Series, Volume II*. Washington, D.C.: Center for Effective Collaboration and Practice, American Institutes for Research.

Wozniak, J.R., White, T., & Schulz, S.C. (2005). Neuropsychological factors in early-onset schizophrenia. In R.L. Findling & S.C. Schulz (Eds.), *Juvenile-onset schizophrenia: assessment, neurobiology, and treatment*. (pp. 125–147). Baltimore, MD: The John Hopkins University Press.

Wright, I. C., Rabe-Hesketh, S., Woodruff, P. W., David, A.S., Murray, R. M., Bullmore, E. T. (2000): Meta-analysis of regional brain volumes in schizophrenia. *American Journal of Psychiatry 157*:16–25.

Yale, PRIME Research Clinic (n.d.). PRIME Research Clinic. Retrieved October 26, 2009 from http://www.med.yale.edu/psych/clinics/prime/prelig.html

Yoshihara, Y., Sugihara, G., Matsumoto, H., Suckling J., Nishimura, K., Toyoda, R., Takei, N. (2008). Voxel-based structural magnetic resonance imaging (MRI) study of patients with early onset schizophrenia. *Annals of General psychiatry, 7*, 1–11.

Yucun, S., Weixi, Z., Lian, S., Xiaoling, Y., Yuhua, C., Dongfeng, Z., Hengyao, S., Entao, S. (1988). A survey of mental disorders in a suburb of Beijing. *International Journal of Mental Health, 16*, 75–80.

Yung, A.R., Killackey, E., Hetrick, S.E., Parker, A.G., Schultze-Lutter, F., Klosterkoetter, J., & McGorry, P.D. (2007). The prevention of schizophrenia. *International Review of Psychiatry, 19*, 633–646.

Yung, A.R., & McGorry, P.D. (1996). The initial prodrome in psychosis: Descriptive and qualitative aspects. *Australian and New Zealand Journal of Psychiatry, 30*, 587–599.

Yung, A.R., Phillips, L., Simons, J., Ward, J., Thompson, K., French, P., & McGorry, P. (2006). Comprehensive assessment of at risk mental states (CAARMS). Melbourne: PACE Clinic, Department of Psychiatry, University of Melbourne, Melbourne, Australia.

Yung, A.R., Yuen, H.P., McGorry, P.D., Phillips, L.J., Kelly, D., & Dell'Olio, M., et al. (2005). Mapping the onset of psychosis: the Comprehensive Assessment of At-Risk Mental States. *Australian and New Zealand Journal of Psychiatry, 39*, 964–971.

Zolkowska, K., Cantor-Graae, E., & McNeil, T.F. (2001). Increased rates of psychosis among immigrants to Sweden: is migration a risk factor for psychosis? *Psychological Medicine, 31*, 669–678.

Zwerling, C., Whitten, P., Sprince, N.L., Davis, C.S., Wallace, R.B., Blanck, P.D., & Heeringa, S.G. (2002). Workforce participation by persons with disabilities: The National Health Interview Survey Disability Supplement, 1994 to 1995. *Journal of Occupational & Environmental Medicine, 44* (4), 358–364.

Index

Breinigsville, PA USA
10 November 2010
249073BV00003B/1/P

9 781441 962713